The NATURAL GUIDE To WOMEN'S HEALTH

Lynda Wharton

MJF BOOKS

NEW YORK

Published by MJF Books
Fine Communications
Two Lincoln Square
60 West 66th Street
New York, NY 10023

Library of Congress Catalog Card Number 95-81600
ISBN 1-56731-095-8

Printed by arrangement with New Harbinger Publications, Inc.

Manufactured in the United States of America

MJF Books and the MJF colophon are trademarks of Fine Creative Media, Inc.

10 9 8 7 6 5 4 3 2 1

We are what we think.
All that we are
arised with our thoughts.
With our thoughts we
make the world.

Speak or act with a pure mind
and happiness will follow you
as your shadow,
unshakeable.

The Dhammapada

For my darling little Rachel
—my special woman of the future . . .
for all you have taught me already

Contents

I would like to thank Peter Waller, Sue Perkins, and Mark Franken for their generous help to a "computer-illiterate."

My deepest gratitude and love go to my very special mother and father, Pat and Bob Wharton, for their constant and unfailing love and support through some difficult times, and for believing that this book would become a reality.

Thanks also to my friends and clients for all their encouragement and support over the past year.

Introduction

As a woman and a health care practitioner, my foremost interest has always been in the health and well-being of women. Most of my practice is made up of women patients from all walks of life, with just as varied an array of health problems. One thing that most of these women have in common is a genuine desire to understand their ill health. They are, almost without exception, interested in understanding their treatment and cooperating with the changes needed to facilitate their return to wellness. However, over time I have come to realize that when it comes to understanding how their own bodies work, women are in general surprisingly ill-informed. Time and time again I see women try alternative therapies as a last resort, after a series of negative experiences with orthodox medicine. Many of these experiences could have been avoided, had the women understood more about their illnesses and their options.

Knowledge is power, and when it comes to health care, a little knowledge can provide a woman with the ability to make informed choices about her own health care. I have written this book with the aim of increasing the awareness of those women who genuinely want to assume more self-responsibility for staying well. Throughout this book, emphasis is on healthy living as a premium health-care investment. The means for returning to full wellness are discussed from a drug-free, holistic (that is, whole person) perspective. I have always acknowledged the importance of orthodox western medicine—indeed, we should all be thankful for the miracles that modern drugs and surgery can perform. At the same time, however, I have been aware of the failings of our allopathic system of health care. In fact, it was this awareness that first prompted my forays into natural health care.

Complementary therapies are becoming increasingly popular and widely accepted by a population that has also become more aware of the deficiencies of the medical mode of treatment. In my practice I hear the same complaints and notes of disillusionment from clients, day after day.

Many of them speak of a seeming indifference on the part of their health care practitioners. In reality the indifference is often the result of time pressures and stresses placed upon each doctor. Patients complain that they are not supplied with adequate information about their health problems, or that the explanation was excessively technical and difficult to understand. The other most common complaint is about the treatment itself. Often patients have suffered debilitating side-effects from medication, or have ended up with a chronic dependence on drugs supposedly prescribed to help them stay "well." More and more, people are questioning this "magic bullet" approach and looking for more all-encompassing solutions to their health problems.

Allopathic medicine is a medicine of the "part," not the whole. The rationale behind this approach is that if you are sick, you will once again be well if you focus on getting rid of the symptoms from that one area of sickness. If, for instance, you have a skin problem, often you will be treated by a dermatologist—a doctor trained specifically to look at the "part" which is the skin. The problem with this approach is that it fails to take into account that humans are more complex than simply a number of separate parts strung together. There is no one part of your body or mind that functions in isolation. What happens in your mind affects what happens in your body, and vice versa. In the same way, what happens in any one organ of your body spills over to affect many other organs and systems. By simply treating symptoms in isolation, there is a risk of completely missing the underlying cause or root of the presenting symptoms. A dermatologist may treat a skin problem with topical applications of cortizone to suppress the symptoms, without ever stopping to consider the deeper causes of the skin problem. For example, skin problems are often the result of stomach and bowel disorders, nutritional imbalances, ongoing stress, and a variety of other internal problems. So instead of remedying the true problem, the client is sent away with a prescription for medication to keep symptoms at bay.

Today, a rapid change seems to be occurring among lay people and medical practitioners alike. They are realizing that true wellness is much, much more than an absence of symptoms. With this awareness comes a questioning and a willingness to assume new self-responsibility. The whole alternative health movement is about teaching people how to *stay* well, through correct living, sound nutrition, exercise, and attaining a state of inner peace. It is also about harnessing and enhancing the self-healing potential that you have within yourself. This is achieved whenever possible without recourse to pharmacological drugs, and with a focus on the whole living organism rather than simply the part manifesting the symptoms—hence the often-used label "holistic" medicine.

Natural Women's Health is in no way intended to replace or interfere with your relationship with your medical practitioner. Remember, allopathic medicine does have many strengths and much to offer. My personal vision has always been to work toward a system of health care where the sole motivation is to provide whichever therapy is of most use to the individual person and the individual complaint. I hope there will come a day when doctors, osteopaths, acupuncturists, homeopaths, and naturopaths can work alongside each other, respecting each other's skills, with a collectively unified vision of providing the best possible health care. Too often today the personal prejudice, ego, and bias of health care practitioners, orthodox and alternative alike, stand in the way of optimum health care for their clients.

The information that follows will teach you the basics of healthy living and provide drug-free solutions to many of the more common female health problems. It is intended to be used in conjunction with the health care offered by professionals in both the allopathic and complementary areas. The list of Further Reading at the back of the book is a selection of some of the more useful women's health books I have come across in my research and will enable you to follow up on a particular area of interest in more depth. Remember that your community's health care services, agencies, and library are useful places to turn for more information about the topics covered here.

Happy reading, and good health to you all!

PART ONE

Staying Well

CHAPTER 1

A Woman's Body—
How It Works

If you are willing to take more responsibility for your own health, you need to be familiar with your body and how it works. Too many women unquestioningly hand responsibility for their health over to doctors, gynecologists, and other health care professionals, without themselves understanding how women's bodies work. Don't let this happen to you. Take the time to familiarize yourself with your own personal landscape, to explore your genitals and your vagina, and to know what your cervix feels like and exactly where it is. You may wish to use a health book such as *Our Bodies, Ourselves* to guide you through your exploration.

A Little Basic Anatomy

The main organ of interest on the outside of your genitals (an area referred to as the vulva) is the little knob of tissue that lies beneath the hood of skin at the top of your vaginal opening, called the *clitoris*. This exquisitely sensitive organ is filled with nerve endings that produce intense sexual excitement when stimulated. The clitoris doesn't perform any particular function other than giving you sexual pleasure.

Just beneath the clitoris, and above the vaginal opening, is the *urinary opening*, through which urine from the bladder is passed. In young women and most virgins the opening to the vagina is partly (or in some rare instances, completely) covered with a thin membrane of skin called the *hymen*. In the past an intact hymen was considered proof of a woman's virginity. It is possible to be a virgin but to have a broken hymen. Bike riding, masturbation, and using tampons can rupture the hymen.

The *vagina* is actually a closed-ended muscular tube about four or five inches long, with an amazing ability to expand to accommodate the largest of penises, or a 12-pound baby! A healthy vagina is a self-controlling environment, able to keep potentially unpleasant bacteria in check by maintaining its slightly acidic pH.

At the upper end of your vagina you can feel a hardish, knob shape—this is the *cervix*, or the neck of your uterus. The cervix has a small opening that allows the passage of menstrual blood out of the uterus, and also allows sperm into the uterus.

Your *uterus* is a hollow organ about the size and shape of an upside-down pear. It has a special, blood-rich lining called the *endometrium*, which thickens throughout the month, and then sheds during your period.

On either side of the upper part of your uterus, there are long, narrow tubes (about four inches long) which extend up into your abdomen. These are the *fallopian tubes*, which allow the passage of the eggs from your ovaries down to your uterus.

The upper part of each fallopian tube ends with little finger-like projections. Suspended a tiny distance below these projections are the almond-shaped *ovaries*. Your ovaries are not actually attached to the fallopian tubes, and when an egg bursts from the ovary every month, these little finger-like projections wave around and entrap the egg to draw it down through the fallopian tube. If the egg meets up with waiting sperm at any point during its four-day journey from the ovary to the uterus, conception occurs. The egg is then embedded in the thick, nutrient-rich

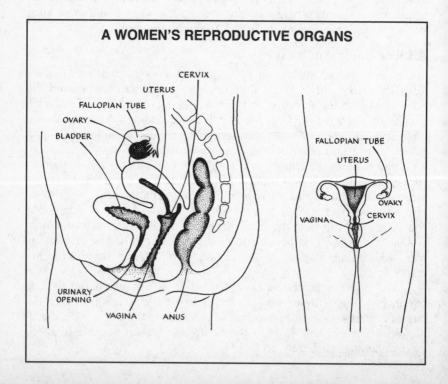

A WOMEN'S REPRODUCTIVE ORGANS

lining of your uterus, and you are pregnant! If your egg remains unfertilized, then your ovaries and pituitary gland (at the base of your brain) begin a complex orchestration of hormones, which ends 14 days later with your endometrium sloughing off as a menstrual period.

Stretching firmly below and around your pelvic organs is a sheath of muscle called the *pelvic floor*. This band of muscle holds all your pelvic organs in place, and provides support for all the other organs in your abdomen, right up to your diaphragm. These muscles cause a multitude of problems if they weaken and fail to perform their task adequately. Pelvic floor repair surgery is an extremely common part of any gynecological hospital's workload. When these muscles weaken, you will probably experience a range of problems, including: poor control of your bladder, with involuntary leaking of urine when you cough, sneeze, laugh, or exercise; inability to empty your bladder fully when you pass urine; a dragging sensation in your lower abdomen, and a feeling that your insides are going to bulge out of your vagina. Indeed, if the prolapse becomes severe enough, this can actually happen. Strong pelvic floor muscles are also important for carrying a baby to term during pregnancy, and for assisting in a normal vaginal delivery. All women are strongly encouraged to perform special pelvic floor strengthening exercises both during and after pregnancy (a condition which itself weakens these crucial muscles), and indeed for the rest of their lives. For detailed information on how to perform these exercises, see Chapter 3 on exercise.

Beginning at Puberty

If you have a young daughter of seven or eight, the last thing that will be on your mind is her eventual development into a sexually and reproductively mature woman. And yet, it is around this age that the very first hormonal stirrings occur which orchestrate this development and the onset of menstruation. At seven or eight your daughter's body is beginning to produce the female hormone estrogen. Over the next few years this hormone will be secreted in ever-increasing amounts, and, along with progesterone, will be responsible for the physiological changes that mark her arrival at womanhood.

Before she begins to menstruate, the pubescent girl will have developed a fairly mature female form—her breasts will have enlarged and the nipples darkened; the external genitals will have enlarged and become thicker and covered with pubic hair; the vagina will become deeper and its walls become thicker; the uterus and cervix will enlarge and the lining of the uterus (endometrium) will have begun its cycle of thickening. The ovaries too will have enlarged, and become more sensitive to the hormones pumped out from the tiny pituitary gland at the base of the brain.

Between the ages of 10 and 16, most adolescent girls will begin their menstrual periods. If your daughter is particularly small or underweight, she will probably be a late starter, as the onset of the menses is largely affected by body weight. The usual weight for the onset of menses is 92 to 102 pounds. For the first two or three years after she begins menstruating, your adolescent daughter will probably experience irregular periods both in terms of onset, duration, and blood loss. This is quite normal and should only cause concern if there is excessive blood loss or pain. It will probably take about 40 menstrual cycles before her particular menstrual pattern is established.

Your Menstrual Cycle

When you were born, your immature ovaries were crammed with around 250,000 eggs, only a handful of which will ever be released, and even fewer of which will be fertilized. From the start of your periods, your ovaries will release one of these eggs each month, continuing this cycle until your reproductive years are over and your menopause begins. As the lining of your ovary bursts and the chosen egg is forced out into your pelvic cavity, the ends of your fallopian tubes move up closer to the ovary and capture the released egg, which then begins its journey down the fallopian tubes to your uterus.

Your uterus is warned by chemical messengers of the impending arrival of the egg, and begins preparing itself for the possible implantation of a fertilized egg. The thick lining of your uterus is further nourished as the blood vessels which supply it with nutrients dilate, increasing the flow of blood to the area. The lining itself doubles in thickness, and is supplied with a banquet of nutrients by the uterine glands.

If this lone egg has been fertilized somewhere along its journey, it will implant itself within this lush lining within three days of arrival in the uterus. If no fertilization and implantation occur, the dilated blood vessels in the uterus return to their normal size. This reduces the nutrient supply to the thickened tissues lining the uterus, and they gradually slough off and pass out of the uterus as a menstrual period.

Most women have a period every 26 to 35 days, with very few sticking to the textbook perfection of a 28-day cycle. As long as your periods are regular, you need not worry unduly about the length of your cycle (unless of course your periods are coming regularly, twice a year!). It is not uncommon for your cycle to become disturbed if you are under a lot of emotional or physical stress, and when you are traveling. Sudden weight loss or gain can also play havoc with your usually regular cycle.

The Four Stages of Your Menstrual Cycle

Your "28"-day cycle is divided into four different stages.

Stage 1 is said to occur from the first day of bleeding, and lasts around five days, until your blood loss stops. Your flow actually contains secretions from your cervix and vagina, tissue from the lining of your uterus, and blood. During your period your ovaries are at their lowest ebb, producing only small amounts of the female hormones, progesterone and estrogen.

Stage 2 of your cycle begins on the day you stop bleeding, and lasts for about 9 days, until just before you ovulate. During this time a tiny gland in your brain (the hypothalamus) nudges your pituitary gland into releasing a particular hormone that sends a strong message to your ovaries. This message triggers some of the eggs in your ovaries to start producing estrogen. Your estrogen levels rise gradually throughout this part of your cycle, reaching a peak around day 13. This high level of estrogen stimulates the lining in your uterus to thicken (in preparation for the imminent arrival of an egg that could be fertilized and ready to implant). The estrogen also causes changes in your breasts and vagina, and you will probably notice an increase in your vaginal discharge.

As well as increasing in quantity, your discharge will also change in quality. By day 13 your discharge will have changed from sticky and creamy to thin, watery, and slippery. Around day 13 of your cycle it will become very stretchy and resemble egg white. This indicates a change in the cellular structure of the discharge—the cells actually realign themselves to make it easier for sperm to pass up through the vagina and

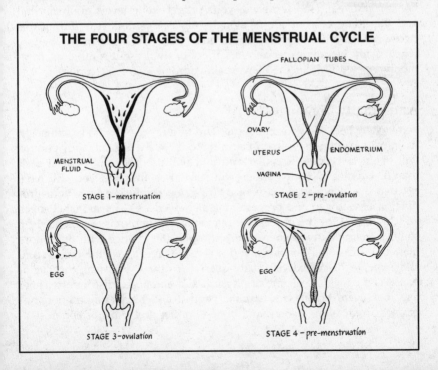

THE FOUR STAGES OF THE MENSTRUAL CYCLE

FALLOPIAN TUBES

MENSTRUAL FLUID

OVARY

UTERUS

ENDOMETRIUM

VAGINA

STAGE 1–menstruation

STAGE 2–pre-ovulation

EGG

EGG

STAGE 3–ovulation

STAGE 4–pre-menstruation

uterus. Your body is out to become pregnant! The discharge also becomes quite alkaline and sugary—in fact, quite nourishing to sperm. You will probably notice a surge in your libido at this time, too, designed by mother nature to make you engage in sex at the time most likely to bring about conception.

Stage 3 occurs when you ovulate, usually around day 14 of your cycle (if you have a 28-day cycle). Just prior to ovulation your estrogen levels peak, causing your pituitary to release another hormone, which in turn causes the egg follicle bulging against the surface of your ovary to burst. Once your egg begins its journey from the ovary, it lives for only 12 to 36 hours. However, because sperm live for up to three (and some people say five) days, you can become pregnant by having unprotected sex three days before you ovulate, or any time in the 36 hours after you ovulate.

Stage 4 begins the day after you ovulate, and lasts until the first day of your bleeding. During this phase your estrogen levels are lower, and your progesterone levels increase and predominate. Your high level of progesterone sends a message to the lining of your uterus, triggering it to secrete nutrients which will be needed should a fertilized egg implant. Even at this pre-conception stage, the progesterone also causes changes in your breasts, in preparation for eventual breastfeeding! You may well notice your breasts becoming swollen and tender at this time.

If your egg isn't fertilized, your progesterone levels gradually fall and the lining of your uterus sloughs off as a period. It is during this two-week duration after ovulation, and before the onset of the period, when many women experience a variety of unpleasant symptoms, commonly labeled PMS or pre-menstrual syndrome (see A-Z section).

And Finally Menopause

Somewhere between your late forties and mid-fifties, your body will begin its transition from its years of being reproductively primed. Your periods will begin to become irregular and you will probably not ovulate each month. Eventually your periods will stop altogether and you will have reached the menopause. As your ovaries stop producing eggs, your production of estrogen and progesterone also decreases—hormonal changes which account for the unpleasant menopausal symptoms experienced by some women. Many women breeze through this change with little more than the occasional hot flash, and a sense of relief that the mess, pain, and expense of periods is finally over! For others, however, the menopause is a bewildering time of physical and emotional discomfort. There may be severe hot flashes, chronic vaginal and bladder infections, migraines, depression, anxiety, and bone-thinning problems (osteoporosis).

Today most women entering the menopause have the option of artificially postponing this natural occurrence through the use of Hormone (or Estrogen) Replacement Therapy (HRT/ERT). This widely promoted and potentially massive source of pharmacological revenue is by no means a perfect form of medication. There are conflicting opinions regarding its long-term safety. The subject of HRT is discussed in detail in Chapter 12.

Breasts and Breast Self-Examination

Your breasts are your other main sexual organ, designed, of course, to nourish and sustain your offspring, but also for many women a zone of intense eroticism and sexual pleasure.

In the center of each breast is the nipple, surrounded by the dark area called the areola. The nipple is made up of erectile tissue which swells and becomes hard when the nipple is stimulated, or in the cold. The interior of the breast is made up of several lobes containing milk-secreting glands surrounded by fat and connective tissue. A network of ducts branches out from the milk-producing glands to the nipple. The whole breast is connected to the muscles of the chest wall by connective tissue.

Your breasts are constantly changing under the influence of your fluctuating hormonal balance throughout the monthly cycle. Every month your breasts are prepared for the possibility of conception and eventual breastfeeding. During the first two weeks of your cycle, the high levels of estrogen in your body stimulate new cells to grow in the glands, milk ducts, and fibrous tissues in your breasts. When you ovulate your body produces more progesterone, which also affects your breasts, this time causing the cells in your breasts to start secreting, and preparing for eventual breastfeeding. At this time you may well notice an increase in your breast size, and tenderness, due to an increase in the amount of blood flowing to the breasts, and also to an increase in fluid retention in your breasts. If you do not become pregnant, your body reverses this breast preparation, slowing down the growth of the new breast cells, and reducing the blood flow to the breasts. These cells and secretions are broken down and reabsorbed by your body.

Getting into the habit of examining your own breasts every month could one day save your life. Breast cancer is one of the most common cancers suffered by women, with one in eleven of us developing this type of cancer at some stage. Over 182,000 new cases of breast cancer (over 500 a day) are diagnosed in the U.S. alone each year. If you check your breasts regularly, you soon become familiar with what is normal and what is not in your own breasts. Many women notice a lot of lumpiness and pain in the second half of their cycle. This is usually caused by fibrocystic breast disease (see A-Z). Although this condition is non-cancerous, it is associated with an increased risk of eventually developing breast cancer;

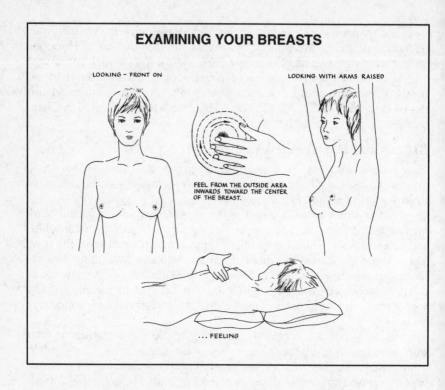

EXAMINING YOUR BREASTS

LOOKING – FRONT ON

LOOKING WITH ARMS RAISED

FEEL FROM THE OUTSIDE AREA
INWARDS TOWARD THE CENTER
OF THE BREAST.

... FEELING

so if you suffer from this complaint, you especially should make breast self-examination (BSE) part of your self-care routine.

It is advisable to begin examining your breasts after your first menstrual period, and certainly by the age of 25 years. Set aside 10 minutes (yes, that's all it takes) on one of the days immediately after your period ends. Your breasts are easier to examine at this time because your hormones are at a low ebb, and consequently your breasts are not swollen or full of fibrocystic lumps. Examining your breasts involves two types of inspection: looking and palpating (feeling).

Looking . . .

Stand in front of a well-lit mirror, with your arms by your sides. Look at your breasts, paying particular attention to their contour. Look for depressions or bulges on the outline of your breasts. Look for dimpling of the skin, and check your nipples for any discharge. Repeat the inspection, but this time with your arms raised above your head. Turn side-on to the mirror so that you can see all areas of your breasts. Check again while you are pushing your palms together in front of you, or standing with your hands pressed against your hips.

. . . And Feeling

For this examination lie down on your back. As you examine your left breast, raise your left arm above your head, with your left hand tucked in under your head and your elbow lying flat against the bed. Using the fatty pads of your fingers, begin to feel your breast gently, beginning on the outside of the breast and working around on the breast in ever-decreasing, systematic circles. Also feel the upper part of your chest wall and the armpit. Repeat on the other side. It is probably easier to feel lumps if you use some kind of lubricant such as body lotion or oil, or perform your examination while you are soaped up in the bathtub.

Remember that when you perform BSE, you are on the alert for any *changes* in your breasts. These changes may not necessarily be lumps. You may detect a sensation of thickening or increased ropiness in your breast tissue, or there may be dimpling or puckering. Whenever you detect an abnormal change in your breasts, see your doctor without hesitation. Ninety-nine times out of a hundred you will have nothing to worry about—and it's worth visiting him or her with a false alarm, rather than delaying action and missing that one-in-a-hundred lump that is cancerous.

If you do find a lump that is diagnosed as cancerous, you will want more information about your situation. The list of Further Reading at the end of the book suggests several publications recommended by the Cancer Society on the subject of breast cancer and its treatment.

Pap Smears—An Important Part of Staying Well

Pap smears are available through your doctor or family planning clinic. They are painless and quick, and there is no valid reason why any sexually active woman should be without them. The pap smear or cervical smear is the most accurate way of detecting abnormal cells that may indicate pre-cancerous changes of the cervix. Before the widespread use of this test, cancer of the cervix was a major cause of cancer deaths in women, largely because the early stages of this cancer are without symptoms.

What Happens in a Pap Smear?

A pap smear involves inserting a small brush (called a cytobrush) into the vagina, where it is gently rotated to pick up some of the body cells that are continually shed by the walls of the vagina and the cervix. These cells are then smeared onto a glass slide, which is sent to a laboratory for analysis.

What Should or Shouldn't I Do Before a Smear?

Your test results are most accurate if you avoid douching for at least five days before your smear. Likewise, avoid spermicidal creams, foams, and jellies for five days before the test. If you have your period, the test cannot be done—you need to have finished your period at least three days before the test.

How Often Should I Have a Smear?

As soon as you become sexually active you should have a pap smear every two years as part of your health-care routine. If you are over 35, an annual test is advisable. If you have a strong family background of cancer, the pap smears can be performed every six months instead.

What Do the Results Mean?

If you have a smear and your results come back *Grade 1*, it means that your smear is completely normal and indicates a healthy cervix.

Grade 2 means that no *malignant* cells were found, but some abnormal cells were found. These abnormal cells usually indicate the presence of an infection and inflammation. Usually you will be advised to have a repeat smear in six months' time.

Grade 3 means that there are warning signs that something is wrong in the way your cervical cells are growing. This result is always followed up with another smear immediately, and a biopsy (where a tiny piece of cervix is snipped away to be analyzed) is usually performed.

Grade 4 means that there are signs of early cancer (technically known as *carcinoma in situ*), which is localized to the area of your cervix or vagina. This result requires immediate follow-up and treatment.

Grade 5 is the most serious abnormal result, indicating invasive cancer. This means that the cancer present in the cervix and vagina is spreading to other parts of the body. This result generally calls for a hysterectomy as well as orthodox cancer therapy such as chemotherapy.

Whatever your results, remember that pap smears are not completely infallible. They can fail to detect abnormal cells if the cell scraping is not performed properly, or due to human error on the part of the laboratory technician classifying the smear. Sometimes a smear may indicate a cancerous or pre-cancerous condition that isn't actually there. This is why any abnormal results are usually followed right away by another smear, to double-check the results.

Chapter 2

Nutrition—
Nourishing the Body

From the moment soon after birth when you first taste your mother's milk, food and eating become firmly implanted in your psyche as one of life's great joys. You eat for pleasure; you eat to share social time with friends; you eat to comfort yourself during times of sadness and depression; and of course you eat to supply your body with the raw materials it needs to regenerate and stay alive.

Strangely, it is this most vital function of nourishment that modern humans often ignore as they pander to the impulses of their tastebuds. People choose the foods that their distorted tastebuds demand—foods that taste sweet or salty, or fat-laden foods that supply rushes of calories. In doing so, people neglect to provide the basic nutrients essential for good health and a long life. Instead, they bestow upon themselves and their children a legacy of "twentieth-century sickness." Cancer, heart disease, obesity, diabetes, and infertility become evermore common health burdens for modern society and individual citizens to bear.

The good news for you and those you love is that with a little nutritional knowledge and application, your health and happiness can be revolutionized. Do you want to feel full of energy and vitality? Do you want to face the challenges of life with excitement and expectation, rather than exhaustion and defeat? Then read on . . .

In general, Americans tend to be overfed, undernourished, and overweight. People consume far too much saturated fat with a high dairy-product and meat intake. They eat too much sugar, too much salt, and too much refined carbohydrate. Consequently, America rates near the top of the tables in the world for incidence of heart disease. Cancer rates are of equal concern, with particularly alarming incidence of cancer of the colon and breast. But you can do your part to turn the health of the nation around virtually overnight by:

- *Decreasing* your consumption of saturated fats, protein, salt, sugar, and refined carbohydrates; and

- *Increasing* your intake of unsaturated vegetable oils, fresh fruits and vegetables, and complex carbohydrates.

Every human being needs the basic building blocks of protein, fats, carbohydrates, and fiber to stay alive. Individual requirements vary greatly, depending upon age, sex, and lifestyle. Pregnancy and lactation also alter your nutritional requirements dramatically. Take a look at some of these nutritional building blocks.

Protein

Protein is a fundamental building block of the human body, accounting for about 20 percent of body weight. It is used to form muscle and bones, internal organs (especially the heart and brain), skin, hair, and nails. Proteins are involved in the production of antibodies, enabling you to fight infection, and many of the hormones circulating in your bloodstream are proteins (including thyroxine and insulin). Americans tend to suffer the ill effects of excess rather than deficient protein intake. Typical sources of protein are animal-based products such as dairy products and meat— foods that supply an excess of harmful saturated fat, along with their protein.

Unlike carbohydrates and fats, proteins are not stored in the body, but must be consumed regularly. Not all proteins are born equal. The building blocks of proteins are chains of amino acids. There are 20 different amino acids in total, 12 of which the body can synthesize itself. The remaining eight amino acids are called "essential" amino acids, and must be supplied through food. Traditionally, the most desirable (and the only, in some people's opinion) source of protein was meat and dairy products. Unfortunately, meat often provides an equal amount of saturated fat (which clogs the blood vessels) along with the protein.

The increasingly popular and healthier alternative is to obtain a fair proportion of your protein from vegetarian sources. Legumes, grains, nuts, and seeds all contain some of the amino acids needed for your body to manufacture protein. Taken in the right combinations, these low-fat, high-fiber foods can supply a complete complement of amino acids. To obtain complete proteins from vegetarian sources, combine grains with legumes, beans, or seeds. For example, eat rice or corn bread or wheat bread with legumes such as beans, lentils, peas, or tofu. Peanut butter on whole grain bread provides a complete protein, as do beans and rice or tofu curry and rice. Soybeans and rice or soybeans with sesame, corn, wheat, or rye also provide complete proteins. Don't forget that nuts and seeds also provide high-quality protein and when used in moderation make a useful addition to the diet—but remember, they also pack a powerful calorie punch!

How Much Protein Do You Need?

Not nearly as much as most of us eat! To work out how much protein you need, multiply your ideal weight (in pounds) by 0.36. This gives you an approximation of your ideal protein intake in grams. If, for instance, your body functions best at a weight of 120 pounds, you need only 43 g of protein a day. In general, women need less protein than men. Growing children (especially toddlers) and adolescents need a relatively high protein intake, as do pregnant and lactating women. As a general rule, pregnant women can multiply their ideal weight (in pounds) by 0.62, and nursing women by 0.53, to find their target daily protein intake in grams.

Fats

Fats are an important source of energy. They are vital for the health of your internal organs, nerves, and cell membranes. They are essential to transport the fat-soluble vitamins (A, D, E, and K) into and around your body. But when it comes to fat, you can definitely have too much of a good thing. There can't be an American alive who hasn't got the message that too much fat is a one-way trip to an early grave. Despite this common knowledge, Americans still obtain more than 40 percent of daily calories from dietary fats—a figure that could do with reducing to the recommended level of 15 percent of calories.

The whole subject of fat and its effect on your health is full of misunderstanding and misinformation for many people. Not all fats are bad for you. Some fats, such as omega-3 fats, are essential for good health. Fats can be broadly divided into two main categories:

- Saturated fats
- Unsaturated fats:
  Polyunsaturated (contains large amounts of Essential Fatty Acids)
  Monounsaturated

Saturated Fats

Animal fats fall into this category. Saturated fats come to you from dairy products (whole milk, butter, and cheese), meat, and meat derivatives such as lard. Coconut and palm oil are saturated vegetable fats. All saturated fats are solid at room temperature. It is these saturated fats that have earned fat such a bad reputation. For a healthier present and future, cut out as much saturated fat as possible.

Unsaturated Fats

Unsaturated fats include polyunsaturated and monounsaturated fats.

Polyunsaturated Fats

You get your polyunsaturated fats from vegetable oils such as safflower, soy, cottonseed, wheat germ, corn, and sunflower oil. Polyunsaturates are often portrayed by advertising companies as your heart's best friend, due to their cholesterol-lowering effect. In fact, the research proving the beneficial effects of polyunsaturated fats on your heart and circulatory system has been inconclusive and confusing. It is true that polyunsaturated oils don't contain cholesterol. There has recently been a change in attitude toward dietary cholesterol. More recent research indicates that the relationship between dietary cholesterol intake and blood cholesterol levels is a lot more complex than previously thought. There does not seem to be a direct correlation between the amount of cholesterol in your diet and the amount of cholesterol in your blood!

It is most important that polyunsaturated oils be kept in the fridge, as they have a tendency to become rancid rather easily. Once rancid, these oils are dangerous and carcinogenic (cancer-causing). Squeeze a couple of capsules of vitamin E oil into your vegetable oils to protect them from oxygenating and becoming rancid.

Omega-3 Fats

Derived from oily fish, this "super oil" was first discovered by scientists researching the low incidence of heart disease among the Eskimo people. Despite their astoundingly high fat intake, Eskimos living in their native environment have one of the lowest incidences of heart disease in the world, thanks to their high intake of omega-3 fatty acids.

You can obtain these cardiovascular protective oils from oily fish such as mackerel, salmon, herrings, grouper, and sardines. By eating as little as three ounces of fish two or three times a week, you can dramatically reduce your likelihood of developing heart disease. Experimental studies have shown a decrease in blood cholesterol levels of around 20 percent within 10 days of beginning a course of supplemental omega-3s.

Essential Fatty Acids (EFAs)

EFAs occur naturally in polyunsaturated vegetable oils, and include linoleic, linolenic, and arachidonic acids. These fatty acids are called "essential" because they must be supplied through dietary sources, as you are unable to manufacture them yourself.

EFAs are essential for your health, and in particular for the growth and maintenance of your blood vessels and nerves, and to maintain the suppleness of your skin and connective tissues. EFAs are also thought to increase the solubility of cholesterol deposits in your arteries, and also to optimize the function of the adrenal and thyroid glands.

Linoleic acid is the most important of the EFAs for you. It is needed for your body to manufacture certain prostaglandins (local hormone-like substances), which are involved in regulating your smooth muscle (that is the muscles which make up many of your internal organs) and the body's inflammatory processes.

SOURCES OF FAT

- Saturated   Beef, chicken, lamb, pork, milk, butter,
                           cheese, yogurt, coconut oil, palm oil

- Polyunsaturated   Soybean oil, safflower oil, sunflower oil,
                           cottonseed oil, corn oil, sesame oil,
                           peanut oil

- Monounsaturated   Olive oil, canola oil, almond oil

- Omega-6 fats   Soybean oil, safflower oil, sunflower oil,
                           corn oil, wheat germ oil, sesame oil

- Omega-3 fats   Flaxseed (linseed) oil, soybean oil, canola
                           oil, pumpkin oil, walnut oil

Because of the common use of chemically extracted oils and a propensity for heating oils during the cooking process, essential fatty acids deficiency can occur. Symptoms of a shortage include a range of skin problems including dryness, scaly skin, or eczema; hair loss; gallstones; slow wound healing; and poor immune function.

Monounsaturated Fats

The most commonly used monounsaturated fats are canola oil and olive oil. These oils are much more stable to heat degradation than polyunsaturated oils, and are suitable for using in cooking (while polyunsaturated fats should really only be used as salad dressings). Monounsaturated oils have been shown to lower "low density lipid" (LDL) levels (the dangerous form of cholesterol).

Margarine and the Polyunsaturate Con

Greater health awareness over the last few years has seen thousands of Americans turn their backs on good old butter in favor of polyunsaturated margarine. Believe it or not, in the butter/margarine debate, margarine is not the goody-goody it once seemed to be. Yes, margarine is made from polyunsaturated vegetable oils, but the process of changing the liquid oil into a solid spreadable product involves bubbling hydrogen through the oil. This process partially saturates the fat, making it no more heart-wise than butter. It also locks away the polyunsaturated fatty acids that were in the original vegetable oil, so your body can't make use of them.

In fact, some research shows that margarine is more damaging than butter for your cardiovascular system. This is largely because margarine contains a high ratio of trans-fatty acids (up to 40 percent in some margarines). These fatty acids decrease the production of certain types of local hormones (prostaglandins), which are responsible for preventing blood clots from forming. Thus excessive intake of trans-fatty acids (margarine) might actually increase the production of blood clots. These same trans-fatty acids also reduce the rate of the conversion of cholesterol into bile salts for excretion. This is the body's way to get rid of cholesterol.

Some margarines also contain many artificial additives and colorings. Your best bet is to keep both butter and margarine use to a minimum.

Cold-pressed Oils—Are They Worth the Price?

When it comes down to choosing your vegetable oils, cold-pressed oils are more expensive than chemically extracted oils, but are worth the extra cost. They contain none of the dozens of artificial chemicals used in the chemical extraction process. The essential fatty acids in cold-pressed oils are unchanged by heat, and are thus more available to your body.

Cold-pressed oils are nutritionally superior to chemically extracted oils, if you intend to use the oil as a salad dressing. If you cook with a cold-pressed oil, you change its chemical bonds in much the same way as has occurred in chemically extracted oils. For this reason you lose some of the benefits of using a cold-pressed oil.

Fats and Heart Disease—A Complicated Story

Everybody knows that too much fat is not good for your heart, but beyond that a host of misconceptions and misinformation abounds. Which fats are good and which are bad? Does having high blood cholesterol mean you'll have a heart attack? How should you lower your blood cholesterol levels? What are triglycerides and how do they affect your health? These are just a few of the questions that are commonly asked.

When it comes to fats and your health, there are two main indicators to consider. One is the total amount of dietary fat you consume. The other is the particular types of fats you consume . . . not all fats are equal when it comes to their impact on your health. While your arteries and blood vessels remain smooth and wide, your blood flows freely and swiftly to nourish and maintain the health of the organs in your body. Over the years, however, the passageways can gradually become caked with fat deposits, which lead to a condition called atherosclerosis. As the resistance to blood flow increases, your heart has to work harder to force the blood through your vessels, and your blood pressure increases. Eventually the increased load on your heart can cause heart disease, angina, and heart attack. It is predominantly the saturated fats (such as dairy products and animal protein) and hydrogenated fats (such as margarine, peanut butter, and most fats used in processed foods) that cause this clogging.

These same saturated fats have been shown to increase your blood cholesterol levels, and elevated cholesterol is known to be *one* of the risk factors for heart disease. High cholesterol levels are especially risky if your blood tests show a high ratio of low density lipids (LDLs) to high density lipids (HDLs). The LDLs are the bad guys when it comes to heart disease. You can manipulate your LDL/HDL ratio through sensible eating and exercise. To decrease your LDLs, simply decrease your intake of saturated fats, and increase your intake of mono- and polyunsaturated vegetable source fats and oils. If you smoke, kick this habit and you will further lower your LDLs. At the same time your HDLs can be increased through regular aerobic-type exercise, and the inclusion of omega-3 fatty acids (especially eicosapentaenoic (EPA) form), which occur naturally in oily fish.

Carbohydrates

Carbohydrates are your source of energy. You burn carbohydrates as fuel to produce energy for life. That piece of bread or serving of pasta you eat is converted into glucose and glycogen to provide energy for your muscles. Carbohydrates fall into two categories—simple and complex carbohydrates.

Simple Carbohydrates

Simple carbohydrates are supplied by sugars—something most people have too much of. Simple carbohydrates are rapidly absorbed in the body, producing a sudden and dramatic elevation of blood sugar levels. These sudden sugar peaks stimulate an equally dramatic outpouring of insulin from the pancreas. It is the job of the insulin hormone to rebalance the blood sugar levels by moving sugar out of the blood and into the cells.

The sense of energy and well-being you feel after your chocolate bar or oatmeal cookie is short-lived and usually followed by an energy crash, a renewed feeling of hunger, and an urge for another sugar pick-me-up. The blood sugar roller-coaster leaves you feeling lethargic and unwell. If allowed to continue for long enough, sugar imbalances may lead to hypoglycemia or "low blood sugar" problems. This syndrome is especially dangerous for individuals with serious metabolic problems such as diabetes. There also seems to be a connection between the amount of simple carbohydrates in your diet and your blood cholesterol levels. As one goes up, so does the other.

Complex Carbohydrates

Complex carbohydrates are quite another story. Also referred to as starches, these more complicated foods are formed by lots of sugar molecules linked together. You get complex carbohydrates from unrefined grains such as whole grain bread, brown rice, whole grain pasta, oats, rye, and vegetables. These "wholefood" carbohydrates are digested and absorbed far more slowly than simple carbohydrates. They provide a gradual, sustained energy source, with none of the attendant dramatic blood sugar fluctuations that occur with more simple sugars.

Complex carbohydrates are satisfying and filling, and more difficult to overdose on. Include plenty of these energy- and nutrient-rich foods in your diet.

A Look at Vitamins and Minerals

Bodies do not live by carbohydrates, proteins, fats, and fiber alone. Without vitamins and minerals, there would be no life; without adequate amounts of these nutrients, there can be no healthy life. The question of what constitutes an "average adequate intake" or "recommended daily allowance" (RDA) is perplexing and at times confusing.

How can you decide upon an "average" desirable nutrient intake when people are all so metabolically unique? Your nutritional requirements change constantly, depending on factors such as emotional or physical stress, ill health, environmental toxins and pollutants, metabolic disorders, smoking, the consumption of coffee and alcohol, use of the contraceptive pill, pharmacological drugs, an unbalanced diet . . . and the list goes on and on. All these unique variables change your individual requirements for particular vitamins and minerals. Consequently, RDAs should be looked upon as no more than very rough, and in many cases inaccurate, rules of thumb.

Do You Need Nutritional Supplements?

Health food shops full of nutritional supplements are a relatively modern phenomenon, and were certainly not on every street corner when your grandparents were young. Your great-grandparents may have lived to a ripe and healthy old age, and not known the first thing about what B complex vitamins could do for them, or how to guard against zinc deficiency. So, do you really need all these cleverly marketed, expensive nutritional supplements?

The answer is not altogether straightforward. Dietary trends have changed so much in the past 60 or so years that it is very difficult to equate the modern diet with that of your grandparents. When bread was all heavy whole grain, and vegetables were eaten in abundance (and grown on soil which was still vital and healthy); when frozen, canned, and processed foods were the exception rather than the rule; when coffee was a rarely sampled luxury, and sweets, chocolates, and cookies were a holiday highlight rather than a daily staple ... when your grandparents were young ... nutritional deficiencies were much less likely.

If you follow the guidelines for building a healthy wholefood diet, the chance of your needing nutritional supplements is smaller than if you survive on a denatured, refined, processed, and unbalanced diet. However, there are times when even the best of diets could do with a little nutritional assistance:

- When you are pregnant and breastfeeding, nutritional supplements are often indicated.

- When you are under a great deal of stress, such as occupational stress, marital disharmony, or the death of someone you love.

- Before and after any kind of surgery.

- If you are chronically ill, or if your immune system often seems to let you down, resulting in frequent colds and flus.

- If you smoke or use the contraceptive pill. (You would be doing yourself a big favor by stopping smoking.)

- If you are on a long-term medication such as tranquilizers, steroids for asthma, or gastric ulcer medication.

If you do fall into one of these groups, and you feel you would benefit from nutritional supplementation, see your health care professional for advice rather than deciding on a willy-nilly cocktail of supplements for yourself. In the long run you will get more value for your money, and avoid unwittingly causing further nutritional imbalances.

The Vitamins

To date about 20 vitamins have been identified as essential for human life. With a few exceptions (such as some of the B complex vitamins), you must obtain these vitamins through food. Vitamins are essential parts of most body enzymes. These enzymes are a part of all the metabolic processes that occur in the body. Consequently, vitamins help regulate the metabolism, help change dietary fat and carbohydrates into energy, and help in the formation of body structures such as bones and tissues.

Vitamins are divided into two main groups:

- Water-soluble, and

- Fat-soluble.

Vitamins C, B complex, and bioflavinoids are water-soluble (that is, they dissolve in water). They are not particularly stable and are rapidly destroyed through the processing and cooking of foods. These vitamins are easily passed out of your body when you urinate. Consequently, they must be replenished daily.

Fat-soluble vitamins such as A, D, E, and K are more readily stored in your body, and consequently they need not be replenished as frequently. They can be stored in fat and in the liver, and drawn on as required. They are not as easily lost from the body as the water-soluble vitamins. However, fat-soluble vitamins have the potential to be more toxic than water-soluble vitamins if taken in excess.

Vitamin B

The B Complex Vitamins

B complex describes a group of water-soluble vitamins that usually occur together in nature. These nutrients need each other for their absorption and utilization to be effective. It is rare to find a particular B vitamin deficiency in isolation. Because of their biochemical interdependence it is generally not a good idea to take any one of the B complex vitamins as a supplement on its own. For example, taking high doses of B_6 without also taking a B complex supplement can lead to a deficiency of vitamin B_2! When you think B complex, think *energy*. Without these vitamins, the body would be unable to change dietary carbohydrates into glucose. You burn this glucose for energy; without B complex vitamins you would be exhausted and listless all the time. If this sounds like an accurate description of you, you would almost certainly benefit from a course of B complex supplements.

Do you have skin problems, thinning hair, a variety of nervous and emotional problems, and mouth sores? Is your appetite poor, and do you dread yet another restless night of tossing and turning in bed? While such symptoms may indicate more serious illness, they may also indicate a B complex deficiency.

What Foods Provide B Complex?

These vitamins are obtained from whole grain (unrefined) cereals such as whole grain bread, whole grain oats, rye, barley, and brown rice. Nuts, leafy green vegetables, and milk are also dietary sources of these vitamins. If you're a meat eater, liver is a B complex power pack. If you're a vegetarian, use brewer's yeast as a tasty supplementary source of these vitamins. Even if you eat a diet rich in these B vitamins, you may still end up with a deficiency if you eat large amounts of sugar, smoke cigarettes, or drink alcohol regularly.

B vitamins are also destroyed by antibiotics, sleeping pills, and the contraceptive pill. If you are under a lot of stress (emotional or physical), or are fighting an infection, your need for B complex increases dramatically. Remember that stress can include pregnancy and lactation. Many female disorders such as pre-menstrual tension, bleeding abnormalities, breast disorders, depression, and minor health problems during pregnancy respond dramatically to supplementary use of B complex.

Vitamin B_1 (Thiamine)

Vitamin B_1 is found in the germ of whole grains. If you eat white bread, you are denying yourself an important source of this vitamin. It can be thought of as the "happy vitamin." Without it, anxiety, neurosis, depression, and behavioral problems soon develop.

If you tire easily, feel irritable and emotionally unbalanced, and tend to have too little appetite, thiamine may be your answer. If you smoke or drink alcohol, or indulge in frequent sugar binges, you will need greater amounts of this vitamin. During pregnancy and breastfeeding, your requirements increase also.

Vitamin B_2 (Riboflavin)

This vitamin plays an essential role in the breakdown of proteins, fats, and carbohydrates. It enhances the metabolism of B_6. Vitamin B_2 is not present in any one food in large amounts, and a deficiency of this vitamin is relatively common.

Sore mouth and tongue and eye problems such as sore, gritty, light-sensitive eyes and cataracts are all symptoms of B_2 deficiency. That red, scaly skin that sometimes develops around your nose, ears, and forehead is also a symptom of a deficiency of this vitamin. If you are pregnant or breastfeeding, or taking the contraceptive pill or Hormone or Estrogen Replacement Therapy (HRT/ERT), then your B_2 requirements are greatly increased.

Vitamin B_3 (Nicotinic Acid, or Niacin, and Nicotinamide)

Like vitamin B_2, B_3 is essential for the metabolism of carbohydrates. It is also essential for a healthy nervous system, and to maintain the health of the skin and the digestive system. This vitamin also improves blood circulation and helps lower blood cholesterol levels.

Vitamin B_3 deficiency is not particularly common. It is usually only seen in people who drink large amounts of alcohol at the expense of their food intake. The symptoms of B_3 deficiency are many and varied. They include skin problems such as dermatitis; weakness and lack of energy; poor appetite and indigestion; and pronounced nervous system disorders such as depression, irritability, tension, and frequent headaches.

B_3 supplements are contraindicated in certain situations. If you are taking medication for high blood pressure, you should speak to your doctor before taking high doses of B3, as this vitamin can cause a substantial drop in your blood pressure. B3 raises blood sugar levels, and so if you are a diabetic you need to use this vitamin under medical supervision. Supplementary niacin seems to have a major contribution in the management of heart disease and problems related to poor circulation, such as muscle cramps, headaches, and Ménière's disease.

Vitamin B5 (Pantothenic Acid)

Pantothenic is derived from the Greek word *Pantos* meaning "everywhere," and indeed this B vitamin is found in a wide range of natural foods. If your diet contains large amounts of whole grains and fresh fruit and vegetables, you can be fairly sure that your B5 needs are being met. This is one of the B vitamins that you can manufacture yourself through the bacteria living in your intestines. That is, presuming that you have healthy intestinal flora that have not been damaged by frequent courses of antibiotics. However, if you depend on white bread, refined cereals, and frozen or canned vegetables as your staples, then watch out. B5 is intimately involved with your metabolism at a cellular level. It is also vital for the release of energy from food.

But first and foremost, pantothenic acid is a supreme stress fighter. This vitamin is essential for healthy functioning of the adrenal glands. These tiny glands, perched on top of each kidney, are a major part of your stress response mechanism. They rarely get a chance to rest as you battle the daily stresses of living in the twentieth century.

If you suffer from abnormal blood sugar fluctuations, chronic fatigue, and an uncomfortable constant aching in the small of your back, your adrenal glands may be trying to tell you something. B5 can improve your ability to withstand daily stress. Your requirements increase dramatically when you are under any kind of ongoing stress, including infection and surgery.

It is also a good idea to use a balanced B complex supplement, including a substantial amount of B5, whenever you are taking antibiotics. This vitamin helps to reduce the toxicity and side-effects of these drugs.

Vitamin B6 (Pyridoxine)

Vitamin B6 is one of the most researched and well known of the B vitamins. It is important for the conversion of energy from all types of food, as well as helping in the production of red blood cells and antibodies. Through its balancing effect on your sodium/potassium ratio, B6 normalizes your fluid balance and is involved in normal electrical functioning of your nerves, heart, and muscles. It is prescribed as a therapeutic supplement in countless doctors' surgeries and naturopaths' clinics every day.

Like vitamin B5, this vitamin occurs naturally in many foods, but is destroyed through the refining and processing of foods. It is quite common to find deficiency states in women who have poor diets, or who go on slimming diets frequently. If you take the contraceptive pill, you should also take a daily balanced B complex supplement containing at least 50 mg of B6.

Serious deficiencies of this vitamin are found in half of all women using the pill. Your need for B6 is markedly increased in any situation where your estrogen levels are increased. This includes the pre-menstrual part of our cycle (and of course during pregnancy), and indeed B6 supplementation is often an integral part of the nutritional treatment of PMS. Used in doses ranging from 50 to 200 mg a day, this vitamin has been proven to reduce breast tenderness, fluid retention, and emotional imbalance associated with PMS. Studies indicate that pregnant women who rely on dietary sources of B6 obtain only about 50 percent of their recommended daily intake—and lactating women don't fare much better, with usual intakes of only two thirds of the RDA.

Since vitamin B6 supplements help so many women with morning sickness, it has been postulated that this condition is partly due to a B6 deficiency, heightened by the high levels of estrogen at this time (which increase your B6 requirements). These results are even more dramatic when you consider that much research indicates that the RDAs of B6 for pregnant and lactating women are far too small anyway. If you are breast-feeding, your milk contains absolutely no B6 until you are taking at least 20 mg of this vitamin each day—that's 1250 percent higher than the recognized RDA of 1.6 mg a day!

Vitamin B6 deficiency during your pregnancy can have more serious repercussions than just making you vomit. It has also been implicated in more frequent occurrence of serious problems in the latter part of your pregnancy, such as toxemia, high blood pressure, and eclampsia. Pregnancy onset diabetes is also more common.

*So How Do You Know if You
Need More B6 in Your Diet?*

Common deficiency symptoms include fatigue, blood sugar fluctuations, fluid retention and pre-menstrual tension, emotional symptoms such as depression, anxiety, and irritability. If you are eating a high protein diet, or a diet high in sugar, your need for this vitamin is markedly increased. The same is true when you are taking antibiotics. If you fall into one of the "high requirement" categories, include plenty of the B6 rich food sources in your diet, as well as using a balanced B supplement supplying at least 50 mg of B6 a day. In most cases B6 supplements are non-toxic, even when taken in large doses. There have been some reports of a type of reversible nerve disorder occurring in people taking more than 250 mg of B6 a day. These reports are rare, however, and all problems were reversed as soon as the supplementation was decreased.

If you take B6 supplements, always take a balanced B complex as well. As is the case with most nutritional supplements, adding large amounts of a certain nutrient in isolation can cause imbalances and deficiency of other nutrients. High doses of B6 taken in isolation can induce a magnesium deficiency. When taking B6 supplements try to ensure that your intake of B1 and B2 are the same as your B6 intake.

Vitamin B9 (Folic Acid or Folacin)

Although this important B vitamin is found in a wide variety of vegetables (in particular leafy green ones), it is easily destroyed in the process of cooking, through exposure to light, and also through storage. Consequently, folic acid deficiency is surprisingly common. It is especially a problem in women taking the pill, or during pregnancy and lactation; in the elderly; in alcoholics; and in people using pharmacological drugs including antibiotics (tetracyclines) and psychiatric medications.

Folic acid is essential for the production of red blood cells, and when deficient, can result in another type of anemia. It has a fundamental part to play in the reproduction and growth of every cell in your body. Obviously then it is especially important that folic acid levels remain high during the time of most cell reproduction—pregnancy (see Chapters 7 and 8 for more information on folic acid).

You could be lacking this vitamin if you suffer from exhaustion, lethargy, lack of appetite, irritability, headaches and a sore or swollen tongue, or anemia. Psychological symptoms include apathy, poor memory and concentration, and irritability.

Folacin is essential for the formation of hemoglobin, the red cells in the blood that carry oxygen. Without sufficient folacin, a type of iron-resistant anemia develops. Although folacin deficiency is not generally very common, there is a very high incidence of deficiency among pregnant women, due to the greatly increased requirements at this time. In fact, when you are pregnant your need for this nutrient doubles.

Folacin is also essential for the formation of nucleic acid, which is needed in great amounts for the rapid production of new body cells which occurs during the growth of a fetus. Today, it is widely acknowledged that there is a strong correlation between a deficiency of folacin during pregnancy and a high incidence of neural tube defects (NTD) such as spina bifida. In one study, several hundred women who had already had one NTD baby were divided into two groups. One group of women received folacin supplements, and the other did not. The effect of the supplements upon the outcome of their next pregnancy was dramatic.

The unsupplemented group had an incidence of NTD babies of 11.5 percent, while in the supplemented group only 0.6 percent of the women had an NTD baby. This translates to a 1900 percent greater incidence of NTD babies in unsupplemented mothers.

Similarly shocking results were obtained in experiments with women who had already had cleft palate and harelip babies. Without supplementation, 7.4 percent of these women went on to produce babies with similar defects—compared with a one percent recurrence in the supplemented group! The message is glaringly obvious. If you are pregnant or trying to become pregnant, optimize your diet ... and use nutritional supplements under the guidance of your health care professional.

Folacin deficiency has also been implicated in toxemia of pregnancy, premature births, and hemorrhaging after birth. Start munching on your three-bean salads and spinach pies!

Vitamin B₁₂ (Cobalamin)

Your body requires only trace amounts of this vitamin, but deficiency in it is a serious—even fatal—condition. B_{12} deficiency rarely occurs, and when it does it usually affects strict vegans who eat no meat, dairy products, or eggs. This is because appreciable amounts of B_{12} are mostly found in animal proteins. If you are a strict vegetarian, your food sources should include spirulina, tempeh, miso, and yogurt containing live *Lactobacillus* bacteria. B_{12} supplements are usually only needed by strict vegans, or in elderly people with absorption problems (in which case the vitamin is administered by injection).

Ongoing lack of B_{12} can result in a particularly nasty type of anemia called pernicious, or megoblastic, anemia. This causes exhaustion and nervous system problems such as weakness, numbness and tingling of the limbs. Left untreated this anemia can be fatal.

Biotin, Choline, and Inositol

Biotin is found in trace amounts in all animal and plant tissues. Particularly good dietary sources include egg yolks, beef, liver, brown rice, and brewer's yeast (yes, again!). Healthy intestinal tract bacteria can also manufacture this vitamin for you. Biotin is important in the metabolism of fat and the production of fatty acids. In therapeutic doses it is often used for skin problems such as eczema or dry, scaly skin.

Choline and inositol are both intimately involved with the health of your cardiovascular system, through their blood cholesterol regulation.

They are also essential for the health of the myelin sheath surrounding each nerve fiber. Choline and inositol are both present in lecithin.

Vitamin C (Ascorbic Acid, Calcium Ascorbate, Sodium Ascorbate)

If this vitamin had been discovered by a pharmaceutical company and its manufacture patented, it would have been marketed as one of the true wonder drugs. The list of indications for the use of vitamin C as a supplement could fill pages. Its use is indicated in any condition of infection, viral or bacterial; any condition of stress, emotional or physical; recovery from surgery; gum problems; skin problems; mental problems; poor immune function; allergies; blood clotting disorders; poisoning; drug addiction. . . .

Humans rate as biochemical oddities when it comes to vitamin C. We (along with guinea pigs and monkeys) are the only species unable to manufacture this vitamin. We are totally dependent upon dietary and supplemental sources. While it is true that vitamin C occurs in many of the fruits and vegetables we eat, it is also true that vitamin C deficiency is surprisingly widespread. (See chart on p. 60 for sources.)

Vitamin C is destroyed by improper storage and cooking of fruits and vegetables. Fruits and vegetables should be refrigerated to conserve maximum amounts of this vitamin. Because it is a water-soluble vitamin, large amounts of C are lost during the boiling of vegetables. Switch to a steamer, and save the water to use as a stock for soups.

Nutritional authorities are still unable to reach an agreement on what constitutes an adequate intake of vitamin C. What is known is that there are several factors that greatly increase your vitamin C needs. Do you smoke? Every cigarette you puff destroys 25 mg of vitamin C in your body. If you are a smoker, you should ensure that your vitamin C intake far exceeds the RDA of 60 mg. If you use steroids regularly, for example, in the control of asthma, skin conditions, or joint injuries and arthritis, make sure that you invest in a bottle of vitamin C. Your requirements are greatly increased. The same applies if you are on a long-term course of antibiotics such as those prescribed for acne. Are you using sulfa drugs, or taking aspirin daily for arthritic pain? You too need vitamin C supplementation.

What Does Vitamin C Do for You?

This wonder vitamin plays a primary role in making and maintaining collagen. This is the protein you use to form all connective tissue in skin, hair, and bones. Without collagen you would look like the baggy, saggy elephant. It may partly explain why women who smoke heavily usually look a good 10 years older than they are. After surgery or injury, such as wounds and burns, you need vitamin C to speed the formation of healing connective tissue. This vitamin is also essential for the formation of red blood cells, and is particularly indicated before any kind of surgery, to reduce the likelihood of hemorrhage. Bleeding gums and easy bruising are two tell-tale signs of vitamin C deficiency, not to be ignored.

Vitamin C has also been shown to increase the ability of white blood cells to fight infection, be it from bacteria or viruses. Megadoses of this vitamin are also used in the treatment of some serious diseases such as cancer and AIDS, with impressive results.

Vitamin C and Pregnancy

If you are pregnant, your vitamin C requirements are increased. Your needs are particularly high in the third trimester, when the growth of the fetus is so rapid. If you develop hemorrhoids during your pregnancy, take it as a clear indication that you need more vitamin C in your diet.

It is not a good idea to take massive doses of vitamin C during pregnancy. Research indicates that if your fetus develops in an overly "C-rich" environment, its post-birth requirements are greatly increased. Women taking 5000 mg of vitamin C a day during pregnancy gave birth to healthy babies who soon developed the symptoms of scurvy (lack of vitamin C).

Vitamin C and Cancer

Vitamin C will not on its own prevent cancer. However, there is a large body of research that indicates that vitamin C does exert some kind of cancer-inhibiting effect. Studies of women with cervical cancer found that they all had lower levels of folacin, beta-carotene, and ascorbic acid than the non-cancerous controls. Likewise, the incidence of pre-cancerous cervical dysplasia was found to be seven times greater in women who regularly consumed less than 60 mg of vitamin C a day, compared with women with a higher nutrient intake.

Some Pointers on How To
Supplement With Vitamin C

Vitamin C supplements are available in several different forms—ascorbic acid, calcium ascorbate, and sodium ascorbate. Although all three types provide the benefits of vitamin C, in some cases one type of supplement is preferable to another. If you suffer from hypertension and follow a low-sodium diet, you are best to avoid the sodium ascorbate form of vitamin C. If you have ever suffered from calcium oxalate kidney stones, you are best to avoid the calcium ascorbate form.

Ascorbic acid can be irritating if you suffer from excessive gastric acid, or gastric ulcers. Use the more gentle calcium form instead. Vitamin C is quickly passed out of the body in urine, so you get more value for your money if you take vitamin C in small frequent doses rather than as one large dose.

If you are using high doses of vitamin C to help fight an acute infection, you may strike what is called "bowel tolerance." Bowel tolerance occurs when you have achieved tissue saturation, and the vitamin C begins to affect your bowels, making your stools loose. This is uncomfortable rather than dangerous. At this stage cut back slightly on your vitamin C intake, until your stools return to normal.

High doses of vitamin C seem to increase your body's expectation and requirements for this vitamin. Consequently, it is important that you reduce your intake gradually. For example, if you have been taking a few thousand milligrams of vitamin C for several days to fight a cold or flu, don't just suddenly stop your supplementation as soon as you feel better. Instead, reduce your intake by a couple of hundred milligrams each day, until you get back down to your usual supplementation rate. Ignoring this advice may set you up for another cold or infection sooner than you had bargained for.

Vitamin C supplements are available as tablets or as a powder that can be mixed with fruit juice to mask the unpleasant taste. Chewable vitamin C tablets have a disastrous effect on your teeth and should be avoided if possible. If you give these pleasant-tasting tablets to your children, make sure they clean their teeth thoroughly right after the tablet. Look for vitamin C supplements that contain bioflavinoids, to enhance absorption (see bioflavinoids below).

Bioflavinoids

Do you carefully peel all the white fleshy pith from your orange and throw it away? If you do, you are throwing away a nutritional jackpot crammed with bioflavinoids. This vitamin, essential for the proper absorption of vitamin C, occurs naturally in citrus fruits, plums, black currants, apricots, blackberries, cherries, and buckwheat. Green peppers, tomatoes, and broccoli are also good dietary sources.

As well as enhancing vitamin C absorption, bioflavinoids perform important functions in their own right. Without adequate bioflavinoids in your diet, your blood capillaries become fragile and rupture easily. The result is easy bruising and bleeding problems such as recurrent nosebleeds, or abnormally heavy menstrual periods. If your monthly periods keep you virtually housebound because of the heavy flow, bioflavinoids (along with other nutritional supplements) may be your key to freedom.

Vitamin A (Retinol or Beta-Carotene)

Vitamin A occurs in two different forms—pre-formed vitamin A (also called retinol, or retinoic acid), which is found in animal tissues, in particular the liver of fish such as cod and halibut; and beta-carotene.

Beta-carotene is the form supplied by fruits and vegetables. It is actually a vitamin A precursor, which is changed into vitamin A in your body. Beta-carotene is found in certain fruits and vegetables, especially the yellow and green range—carrots, apricots, broccoli, and spinach.

What Does Vitamin A Do for You?

When you think of vitamin A, think of your eyes, skin, and mucous membranes (such as the lining of the lungs, mouth, stomach, vagina, etc.). This vitamin is essential for the health of your skin, and without enough of it, your covering becomes rough, dry, and covered with acne! Your inner linings also rely on vitamin A for their health. By strengthening the walls of the cells in the mucous membranes such as the lungs, this vitamin improves your resistance to invading bacteria.

You can see in the dark thanks to vitamin A. If you find night driving difficult because you are blinded by oncoming headlights, then you have a clear indication that you need more of this vitamin in your diet. Like vitamin C, vitamin A (in particular beta-carotene) has been proven to have cancer-preventing qualities. Women with low intakes of vitamin A are very much more at risk of developing cancer of the endometrium or cervix than women with higher vitamin A intake. This protective effect results from beta-carotene's ability to soak up the "free radicals" (unstable molecules) that are partly responsible for the creation of deviant cancer cells.

Your immune system is also stimulated by beta-carotene, thus increasing your ability to destroy deviant cells before they multiply to form cancer.

Do you have horrific childhood memories of a compulsory daily dose of foul-tasting cod liver oil? Despite tasting like poison, your mother was doing you a great favor with her home remedy. Fish liver oil is the richest source of pre-formed vitamin A.

When it comes to using vitamin A supplements, there are differences between pre-formed vitamin A and beta-carotene. Pre-formed vitamin A can be toxic when taken in excess for long periods of time. It is inadvisable to take more than 20,000 iu daily without some professional guidance.

Beta-carotene, on the other hand, can be taken in massive doses without any danger of toxicity. However, beta-carotene is not a suitable supplementary source for everyone. If you have diabetes or a sluggish thyroid, your ability to transform beta-carotene into usable vitamin A is greatly reduced. Try to increase your natural intake of beta-carotene rather than (or as well as) relying on nutritional supplements.

When it comes to vegetables and beta-carotene, cooked is better than raw. Cooking, chopping, and mashing increases the absorbability of this vitamin. Vitamin A absorption and utilization are also enhanced by the mineral zinc, so if you're low in zinc (an alarmingly common condition), then you're also likely to have problems making use of your ingested vitamin A.

If you're using large amounts of supplemental vitamin A (upwards of 50,000 iu a day) watch out for symptoms of vitamin A toxicity. These include frontal headaches (due to a slight swelling of the brain), nausea and vomiting, irritability, dizziness, and hair loss. Your skin may itch and become flaky and you may lose your appetite. These signs of "hypervitaminosis" are all reversible when you reduce your intake of the vitamin.

One more word of caution—if you are pregnant or planning to become pregnant, limit your supplementation with pre-formed vitamin A (retinol) to no more than 15,000 iu a day. Some research suggests that higher doses can cause fetal abnormalities. However, you can supplement with large amounts of beta-carotene without risk to your child or yourself.

Vitamin C (Calciferol)

Vitamin D is one of those vitamins (like some of the B complex) which you can manufacture yourself, with the aid of the sunlight upon your skin. The "sunshine vitamin" is essential for the proper absorption and utilization of calcium, and is essential for the normal calcification of bones.

The old scourge of the lower classes during the Industrial Revolution was rickets—the bone-deforming disease resulting from a lack of sunshine and dietary vitamin D. Vitamin D requirements are increased during pregnancy and breastfeeding, and also during the menopause when calcium absorption and utilization changes, due to the decline of estrogen production. Infants and children with rapidly developing skeletons also need greater amounts of this vitamin.

Sunshine aside, you can obtain vitamin D through food sources such as egg yolks, liver, and fish. Milk is also enriched with vitamin D. Because of your ability to manufacture this vitamin, vitamin D deficiency is relatively rare these days, and only a problem for elderly people, as their skin production tends to be lower (and they are often exposed to little sunshine).

Bowel problems such as ulcerative colitis also reduce your ability to absorb this nutrient from food.

Vitamin E (Tocopherol)

Vitamin E is another of the "super nutrients" (like vitamin C) that have been researched and written about in abundance. Despite the huge body of evidence proving very many therapeutic uses for this vitamin, few people obtain adequate amounts from food alone. It is most richly supplied in cold-pressed vegetable oils, raw nuts and seeds, soybeans, and the germ of whole grains . . . none of which are staples of the average Western diet. Look in most supermarket carts at the mountains of white bread and commercially denatured cooking oils and you will see why so few have their requirements for this vitamin met. Adding more vitamin E to your diet is as simple as changing to a whole grain bread, and including a teaspoon of cold-pressed oils in your diet each day, in particular wheat germ and safflower oil. Sprinkling fresh wheat germ on your hot or cold cereal in the mornings also supplies a delicious powerpack of vitamin E.

What Does Vitamin E Do for You?

The therapeutic claims for this vitamin are almost endless (and in some cases quite contentious), but there are certain proven functions for this vitamin. Vitamin E is an anti-oxidant (along with vitamin C, beta-caro-tene, and selenium), which means that it is able to protect your body cells from destruction by preventing them from reacting with oxygen. These internal oxygen molecules are given the delightful name of "free radi-cals." Their name may be poetic, but their effects on your health are far from amusing. Free radicals contribute to the development of a range of nasty degenerative illnesses such as atherosclerosis, high blood pressure, heart disease, arthritis, and cancer, and premature aging in general.

It is this anti-oxidant effect that has earned vitamin E its reputation as the "youth vitamin." Vitamin E is the vitamin par excellence when it comes to circulatory or heart disorders. It is a natural, non-toxic blood thinner, preventing clots from forming in the blood and breaking away to cause strokes or heart attacks. Because of this anti-clotting effect, it is unwise to take large amounts (more than 300 iu a day) of supplemental vitamin E before undergoing surgery or in the weeks leading up to child-birth. Taken in smaller doses this nutrient will assist with healing after surgery and reduce the likelihood of post-operative problems with blood clots.

Vitamin E also helps your muscle cells to breathe. Generous supplies of vitamin E allow muscle cells to function effectively on smaller amounts of oxygen. This adds up to a noticeable improvement in energy levels, endurance, and stamina. Applied topically to scars and wounds, vitamin E can work miracles. If you have a scar or adhesions from surgery, pierce a vitamin E capsule and apply the oil twice daily for several weeks. You'll be amazed at how the adhesions soften and the scars fade.

Women and Vitamin E

Vitamin E has been used successfully to treat a wide variety of female problems, including irregular periods, scanty periods, painful periods, itching and inflammation of the vagina, and hot flashes experienced dur-ing the menopause. When it comes to period pain, vitamin E is nature's alternative to prostaglandin inhibitors such as aspirin. Your uterus produces local hormones called prostaglandins, an excess of which are partly responsible for overly fierce uterine contractions during your period. Non-steroidal anti-inflammatories such as aspirin or mefenamic acid (Ponstel) slow down (or stop) the production of these prostaglandins, thus greatly reducing menstrual pain. Vitamin E is nature's alternative to these drugs, with its ability also to reduce these same local hormones. It also helps ease pain by enhancing circulation, and reducing the amount of oxygen needed by working muscles.

During your period, the powerful muscle of the uterus contracts dramatically, forcing out the menstrual blood. It is thought that it is this powerful contraction, and the resulting constriction of blood supply to the uterus, that causes the pain of menstrual cramps. Vitamin E enhances blood supply to the uterus, and at the same time reduces its oxygen requirements, thus lessening pain.

Thanks to vitamin E, there is no reason why any menopausal woman should continue to suffer the annoyance and discomfort of hot flashes. Supplements will often also help alleviate the vaginal thinning and itching that accompanies the decline in estrogen production (see Chapter 12 on menopause).

Some Hints About Using Vitamin E Supplements

Vitamin E supplements come in d (one molecule) and dl (two molecule synthetic) forms, of which the natural d-alpha tocopherols are the most potent and best value for the money. As most vitamin E supplements are oil-filled capsules, they should be refrigerated after opening to help prevent rancidity. Vitamin E supplements are best taken before breakfast or before going to bed, or after meals containing some fat.

Besides the health problems already discussed, there are certain other situations where vitamin E supplements are appropriate. If you take the contraceptive pill or HRT/ERT, you might consider vitamin E supplementation, as estrogen interferes with the absorption of this vitamin. Your need for this vitamin increases as your intake of polyunsaturated fats increases.

If you use a lot of vegetable oil in cooking or salad dressings, you will need to increase your intake of vitamin E. Vegetable oils increase the rate of destruction (oxidation) of vitamin E. It is also a good idea to use vitamin E supplements if you are taking large amounts of evening primrose oil as a supplement. If you are taking iron supplements, and especially if they are inorganic iron (which is usually prescribed by doctors for pregnant women), take your vitamin E eight to 12 hours before or after the iron. These two substances hinder each other's absorption.

If you plan on using large amounts of vitamin E (for example, 400 iu or more daily) for therapeutic purposes, do so under the supervision of your health professional. This vitamin can cause problems in some people if taken in excess. For example, anyone with high blood pressure should introduce vitamin E in gradual stages, as too much given too quickly can cause an increase in blood pressure. If you are on pharmacological blood-thinning drugs, the addition of vitamin E without your doctor's knowledge could lead to dangerously thinned blood, with resultant hemorrhage.

The Minerals

Minerals, like vitamins, are essential for life. Human bodies tolerate a lack of minerals less effectively than they can tolerate vitamin deficiency, and yet people are more commonly lacking in minerals than vitamins. This is partly because minerals are harder to digest and absorb, and there is a lot more competition between minerals for absorption. For example, large amounts of zinc will reduce your absorption of iron, copper, and phosphorus, while too much calcium (usually in supplemental form) hinders your uptake of magnesium, zinc, and manganese. You must obtain all the minerals you need from food, as your body is unable to manufacture them. Minerals come to you through the food chain, from the earth. When the soils are depleted and lacking vital minerals, food becomes a correspondingly poor source of minerals. Organically grown produce is one alternative that emphasizes growing conditions suited to a rich transfer of vitamins and minerals from the earth to you.

Calcium

Of all the essential minerals, calcium is needed in the greatest abundance. Without calcium, your bones would crumble and your teeth would fall out; your nervous system would be in tatters and your muscles would be useless.

This mineral is essential for building and maintaining a strong break-resistant skeleton. The one percent of body calcium that circulates in your bloodstream (as opposed to being locked within your bones) is responsible for muscle contraction and relaxation—calcium deficiency is a very common cause of muscle cramps. Blood calcium is also essential to regulate the pH of the blood, and to assist with blood clotting whenever necessary.

Whenever you think of calcium sources, you always think of dairy products first. And yes, it's true, dairy products do contain large amounts of calcium. But this dietary supply is not suitable for everyone. Dairy products tend also to supply large amounts of saturated fats. Dairy intolerance is also quite common, especially among children. Even among people who are not allergic to dairy products, large amounts of milk and cheese can be very mucus-forming.

There are other useful dietary sources of calcium, such as green vegetables (broccoli, kale, watercress); tempeh and tofu (fermented soybean products); bony fish such as sardines, pilchards, salmon, and herrings; and almonds. Even with generous dietary supplies of calcium, bodily absorption is usually quite poor. In fact, you absorb only about 20 to 30 percent of what you consume. Your absorption will be especially poor if you have trouble with low stomach acid, or if you frequently use antacids or ulcer-type medications such as Zantac.

If you eat a high-fat diet, or if you are deficient in vitamins A and C, or D, your calcium absorption will be inefficient. Excesses of certain types of food in your diet can also interfere with your absorption of this important mineral. These include foods containing large amounts of oxalic acid, such as spinach, rhubarb, and chocolate.

Whole grains contain phytic acid, which also tends to reduce absorption of calcium and other minerals. Too much salt or sugar causes you to lose more calcium in your urine. The contraceptive pill affects your body chemistry in a myriad of ways, one of which is the lowering of your blood calcium levels. No amount of calcium supplements will fully compensate for this drop in blood calcium level.

How Do You Know if You Are Calcium-Deficient?

There are certain common warning signs that indicate you could do with more of this mineral. Do your muscles seize in painful cramps? Does your heart sometimes race out of control, for no particular reason? Does your family accuse you of being a nervous wreck—tense and flying off the handle with the least provocation? Maybe your teeth feel loose, or keep you running back to the dentist for yet more fillings. If this sounds like you, then calcium foods and supplements would be a good idea.

Another more sinister indication of calcium deficiency takes years to manifest, and is difficult to put right once it occurs—osteoporosis.

Calcium and Women's Problems

Calcium supplements are used as a part of the treatment for a variety of gynecological disorders including painful periods, menopausal hot flashes, and the emotional turmoil that often accompanies the menopause (see dysmenorrhea in A-Z, and see Chapter 12 on menopause).

Some Tips About Calcium Supplements

Walk into a chemist or health food shop looking for a calcium supplement, and you will be greeted by a bewildering variety. Without some inside information, you could well end up wasting your money. The most common supplementary sources of calcium are:

- Calcium orotate
- Calcium lactate

- Calcium citrate
- Hydroxyapetate
- Calcium carbonate
- Oyster shell
- Dolomite
- Bonemeal

Of these the first four are the most absorbable, and consequently the best value for your money.

Hydroxyapetate is one of the more recently available supplementary forms of calcium, and one which is particularly useful (despite being a little more expensive than the others). Hydroxyapetate is the form it actually takes inside your bones, which is why this form is the most effectively absorbed.

Next in line comes calcium citrate, which is particularly useful for post-menopausal women and for anyone with low stomach acidity. It is also a good choice for anyone who has had trouble with calcium oxalate kidney stones, as it has been proven not to contribute to their formation.

Refined calcium carbonate products have the advantage of being available in a form compounded with vitamin D, which is necessary for calcium absorption, and they also have a very low lead content. However, the high calcium content and the lower assorption rate of carbonate products make them a poor choice for anyone with low stomach acidity.

The last three types of calcium are poorly absorbed. Bone meal and dolomite can also be contaminated with toxic heavy metals such as lead. Dolomite is literally ground up mountains—anyone can work out that human bodies are not designed to digest mountains!

Make sure that the supplement you use is balanced with other vitamins and minerals essential for the absorption and utilization of calcium—most importantly, vitamin D, magnesium, and phosphorus.

Calcium supplements are best taken on an empty stomach, as they need a highly acidic environment to be absorbed. Take your supplements with a little fruit juice to further enhance absorption. Just before bed is a good time to take this supplement; not only will the calcium ensure a great night's sleep, but it will compensate for the large amount of calcium you lose in the first urine of the morning.

Although calcium supplements are often useful, like all good things, it is possible to overdo it. Calcium can be toxic when taken in excess—that is, more than 4000 mg a day (which is an awful lot of calcium). Taken at these doses, calcium can precipitate out of your blood, causing problems with abnormal deposits in your muscles and soft tissues.

Calcium supplements may also cause problems if you have had a history of calcium oxalate kidney stones. However, both of these problems can be easily overcome by using the calcium citrate or hydroxyapetate form of supplements.

Magnesium

Ideally, magnesium is supplied from fresh green vegetables. However, vegetables can only give you the magnesium that they have absorbed from the soils in which they grew—and that's where the problem is! In areas where soils are lacking in this essential mineral, magnesium deficiency is very common. As you'll see, this problem comes up with other minerals, too, such as zinc and iodine.

Magnesium also abounds in raw, unmilled wheat germ, soybeans, figs, corn, and oily nuts and seeds. With the exception of corn, these foods are not staples in the average American diet. Low magnesium intake is further sabotaged by chopping and cooking, processes that destroy what little magnesium the foods contain. Meanwhile, frequent cups of tea and coffee, and a little too much alcohol and sugar, all increase your magnesium requirements. If you have liver, intestinal, pancreas, or kidney disease, your absorption of magnesium will be especially poor.

You need magnesium in your cells for the production and transfer of energy. Magnesium is essential for the synthesis of protein, and for the proper functioning of your nerves and muscles. It is nature's muscle relaxant and an anti-stress mineral supreme. It also helps you to absorb other minerals, such as calcium and phosphorus, and vitamins B, C, and E.

You can suspect a magnesium deficiency if your nervous system feels shot to pieces—if you jump every time the phone rings, and all those advertisements screaming at you from the television make you feel like screaming, too. If you have ever experienced that sensation of muscles in your eyelids twitching, it is usually due to a lack of magnesium.

Inexplicable depression often responds well to calcium and magnesium supplements. These minerals are also used effectively for pre-menstrual tension. Lack of appetite, insomnia, poor memory, general apathy, and rapid heartbeat are all other common symptoms of lack of magnesium.

Magnesium should not be taken as a supplement in isolation, as it can upset the balance of other minerals, in particular calcium. If you need to take supplemental magnesium, use a balanced multi-mineral formula.

PMS, Menstrual Cramps, and Magnesium

Several clinical studies have shown that women with PMS usually have low levels of magnesium. If you go to your doctor complaining of PMS, he or she will probably give you a bottle of B6 tablets. While it's true that B6 can theoretically help you with your symptoms of depression, anxiety, and bloating, it can only work if you have adequate magnesium levels in your body. Magnesium is needed for your body to convert your B supplements into a form that it can use.

Magnesium deficiency also contributes indirectly to uncomfortable pre-menstrual (or even month-long) bloating. The brain neuro-transmitter dopamine needs magnesium to function. When dopamine levels are low, the adrenal hormone aldosterone, which controls the body's water levels, rages out of control. Too much aldosterone causes edema and bloating. Magnesium (along with calcium) can work miracles on period cramps.

Calcium is essential for the proper contraction of muscle fibers, and magnesium in turn is needed to relax these muscle fibers. Magnesium deficiency leads to cramps of all sorts, including uterine cramps.

A Word on Supplementation

As is the case with all other mineral supplements, not all forms of magnesium are equal in terms of absorbability and value for the money. The most easily absorbed forms include magnesium chelate, magnesium aspartate, and citrate. The bicarbonate, oxide, or carbonate forms are less absorbable. Taking magnesium supplements with your meals will reduce your hydrochloric acid production and slow the digestion of your meal as well as the absorption of your mineral supplement.

Take calcium and magnesium supplements on an empty stomach, along with a little ascorbic acid to maximize absorption. Just before bed is a good time to take them, and the natural, soporific effect of magnesium and calcium will ensure a peaceful, deep sleep.

Potassium

This electrically charged mineral is found inside your blood cells, and along with sodium is classed as an "electrolyte." In fact potassium and sodium have a special relationship, and must be finely balanced for good health. The combination of potassium and sodium maintains a normal balance of fluids in your body, and prevents fluid retention, edema, and an increase in blood volume, which can cause hypertension. Potassium is also important for normal muscle contraction and a regular heartbeat.

Because potassium occurs in a wide range of natural foods, our ancestors need not have worried about obtaining adequate potassium from their daily diet. They existed on a wholefood, unrefined diet, low in sodium and abundant in fresh fruits and vegetables (high potassium).

Today, however, things are different. Not only has industrial society turned the natural high potassium/low sodium ratio on its head, but today's diet abounds in denatured, processed, and potassium-depleted foods. Now we binge on a multitude of high-sodium foods (salt in any form, potato chips, snack foods, frozen and canned foods with added salt, cheese, etc.), and have little in the way of fresh fruit, vegetables, and whole grains to supply the balancing potassium you need. This situation of excess sodium to potassium leads to fluid retention, edema and heart problems, and often a prescription for diuretics (which only worsen the situation in the long run by further depleting your potassium stores).

Even if your diet is rich in potassium foods, you may need additional supplies during heatwaves when you lose a lot of potassium in your sweat; after a bout of diarrhea or vomiting; or if you use drugs such as diuretics, laxatives, aspirin, digitalis, or cortisone.

Early symptoms of a lack of potassium include chronic fatigue, weak muscles, slow reflexes, and skin problems such as dry skin or acne. This is usually quickly remedied by reducing the amount of salt in your diet, and increasing your intake of fresh raw fruits, vegetables, and juices.

Sodium

Modern diets are drastically overloaded with this essential (but in excess damaging) mineral. Like potassium, sodium has an electrical charge, making it an electrolyte. It is found mostly in the fluid surrounding blood cells (extracellular fluid), and is intimately involved in the regulation of body fluid. In a nutshell, excess sodium (usually along with insufficient potassium) tends to cause retention of fluid, increased blood volume, and increased blood pressure. This is one mineral with which your concern should not be with ensuring sufficient supplies, but rather with trying to cut down on your intake.

Iodine

Iodine differs from the other minerals discussed so far, in that it is needed in only trace amounts to maintain health. If these trace amounts are lacking, a number of health problems arise, particularly with the function of the thyroid gland, situated at the base of the throat. You need iodine for your thyroid gland to produce the hormones that regulate your metabolism and set your basal metabolic rate.

Iodine deficiency is rarely a problem these days, as most table salt is enriched with iodine. Although many soils lack this trace element, iodine is also supplied through seafoods such as fish, shellfish, and seaweed. Kelp is the form of iodine most commonly used as an iodine supplement. Indeed, eating kelp or kelp tablets is a good way of ensuring adequate iodine intake if you are a vegetarian (that is, don't eat seafoods), and use little or no salt. As with all good things, though, you can overdo it. Excessive intake of iodine, in the form of mountains of kelp tablets for example, has been shown to reduce the production of thyroxine and cause sluggish thyroid function.

If your thyroid gland is failing to obtain sufficient dietary iodine, it can react in a number of ways. Probably the most visually dramatic is the development of goiter, which is an enlargement of the gland and the whole neck. This problem was especially common in America in the 1930s and 1940s, in the midwestern states where the soil lacked iodine.

In other cases iodine deficiency results in a condition of hypothyroidism, or sluggish thyroid function. This condition causes weight gain, lethargy, poor temperature regulation (with a feeling of constant cold), dry skin and hair, and mental symptoms such as depression and apathy. There are often also menstrual problems such as irregular or absent periods or excessively heavy periods.

Iron

Many of those growing up in the 1960s and 1970s experienced the very dubious honor of courses of iron tonics when mothers thought their children looked a little too pale. Ghostly complexions and lack of energy and stamina have long been recognized as the clearest indications of iron deficiency anemia. The inorganic iron supplements that children were fed, and that some women are still given during pregnancy, are not the best way of dealing with iron deficiency. These ferrous sulphate tonics can be toxic, are poorly absorbed, and often cause terrible constipation.

If you suspect that you need more iron, there are some simple dietary changes that you can try before resorting to supplements.

Why Do You Need Iron?

Iron is the main blood mineral. It is essential for the formation of hemoglobin (the red pigment in your blood), which is responsible for delivering oxygen to your body tissues. Without iron your muscles and cells are deprived of oxygen, and you feel the results as lethargy, breathlessness, and fatigue. Without adequate iron, your brain also suffers from lack of oxygen. If your short-term memory is terrible, and your concentration feeble, you may be lacking in iron. Dizziness and frequent headaches are other warning signs. Your fingernails can indicate your iron status, too. If they are brittle and flattened (or even worse, spoon-shaped) and covered with longitudinal ridges, you need more iron in your diet.

Iron deficiency is most commonly a female problem, because of the ongoing loss of blood (and the iron it contains) through the monthly periods.

How Can You Get More Iron From Your Diet?

You can start by increasing your intake of iron-rich foods. Red meat (and in particular liver and other organ meats) is the most abundant and efficiently absorbed source of iron. Of course, you'll want to keep an eye on fat intake with these animal sources, selecting the leanest cuts possible. Vegetarian sources include green leafy vegetables (providing that they are grown in iron-rich soil, and have a lovely dark green coloring), cherries, apricots, plums, grape juice, dried fruits, legumes such as peas and lentils, molasses, brewer's yeast, and wheat germ.

Eat a good vitamin C source along with your iron-rich foods to enhance the iron absorption—for example, chopped tomatoes along with your green leafy vegetables, or a glass of freshly squeezed orange juice with your meals. Do you usually sit down for a cup of tea or coffee straight after a meal? This practice greatly hinders your iron absorption from the food you have just eaten. Wait at least an hour before you indulge.

Iron Supplements

It can take up to six months of a new iron-rich diet before you feel the benefits. There are times, however, when dietary enrichment alone is not enough; for example, during pregnancy and breastfeeding, or following heavy blood loss such as childbirth or surgery. At these times it is a good idea to use a balanced iron supplement, with professional supervision.

Iron can be toxic when taken in excess, and it is never a good idea to self-medicate for long periods of time. However, having determined your genuine need for an iron supplement, there are a few things you need to know. I personally have found two iron formulas in particular to be especially useful and safe. These are the Floradix iron tonic and Bioforce. Floradix is an organic, yeast-grown iron, balanced with vitamin C-rich fruit extracts (to enhance absorption) and B complex vitamins. This effective formula has extremely low toxicity and is especially useful for recovery from surgery, during pregnancy, postnatally, and also for children. Bioforce is similarly useful, but is perhaps more appropriate than Floradix for women suffering from candida or yeast intolerance problems.

Any iron supplements should be taken on an empty stomach (because of the large amounts of stomach acid needed to absorb iron), and well away from any vitamin E supplements you may be taking. Leave at least eight to twelve hours between taking vitamin E and iron, as they interfere with each other's absorption.

Zinc

After iron, zinc is the trace mineral you need most of. You can obtain sufficient zinc from a wholefood diet rich in whole grains, nuts, seeds (especially pumpkin seeds), and some red meat. However, vegetarians who are denied the most abundant supplies of zinc (animal flesh and seafood) often develop symptoms of zinc deficiency, despite their high intake of whole foods. This is partly because many soils are lacking in this trace mineral, and consequently, so are their grains and vegetables. Processing and cooking of foods also destroys what zinc is present. Vegetarians are more likely to be zinc-deficient for other reasons too—the zinc bound with phytates and oxalates present in grains and vegetables is poorly absorbed, compared to animal protein sources. High-fiber foods also tend to inhibit zinc absorption. (That doesn't mean you should cut out the fiber!)

Other useful sources of dietary zinc include herrings, oysters, liver, mushrooms, wheat germ, onions, and good old brewer's yeast. Dietary zinc sources need to be a regular part of your diet, as you are unable to store zinc for times of increased need.

Pregnancy and lactation increase your zinc requirements dramatically, as do taking the contraceptive pill, repeated weight-loss diets, and drinking alcohol regularly.

Zinc is needed for nearly all metabolic functions. It is an integral part of the formation of hormones such as insulin. It is essential for proper growth and development, especially of the reproductive organs. Zinc is needed to heal wounds, and for your immune system to fight infection.

Signs of zinc deficiency include frequent infections, skin problems such as acne or stretch marks, blood sugar problems, little white flecks on your fingernails, thinning hair, and a poor sense of taste. Zinc-deficient teenage girls are usually very late in beginning menstruation. When they do start menstruating, their periods are often irregular.

Zinc and Pregnancy

If you are low in zinc when you conceive, and during the months of your pregnancy, you increase your likelihood of developing a range of unpleasant problems. Zinc-deficient pregnant women are at greater risk of developing hypertensive problems such as edema, toxemia, and eclampsia. On a purely cosmetic note, you also predispose yourself to developing unsightly stretch marks which will stay with you for life. Your baby suffers too, and is more likely to be born underweight and unhealthy.

If you are taking iron supplements during your pregnancy, and your diet is low in zinc, you are almost certain to be zinc-deficient. Iron competes with zinc for absorption, and so supplemental iron can further decrease your zinc status. The recommended daily intake of zinc for pregnant women is 15 mg, and since most women studied are found to have intakes of no more than 10 mg a day, a zinc supplement during pregnancy is probably a good idea. Seek professional advice rather than formulating your own cocktail of nutritional supplements.

A Note on Supplementing With Zinc

If you are a vegetarian, pregnant, lactating, or growing quickly (early childhood and adolescence), you may well need additional supplementary zinc. In terms of supplements, chelated zinc is usually the best tolerated and most efficiently absorbed (as well as the most costly!) form of zinc. You can further enhance your absorption of this mineral by taking your supplement on its own two hours after your meals, or first thing in the morning.

As with all the other nutrients discussed in this chapter, simply taking large amounts of this mineral in isolation can cause deficiency prob-

THE IMMUNE BOOSTER PROGRAM

- Vitamin A — 10,000 iu
- Vitamin E — 400-600 iu
- B complex — Supplying 50 mg of the major B vitamins
- B_5 — Additional B_5, up to 500 mg
- Vitamin C — 2000-5000 mg
- Multi-mineral — Containing zinc, iron, selenium, calcium, and magnesium, in orotate or chelate form

Certain herbs are also useful to guard against infection when taken regularly. The most common include:

- Garlic
- Echinacea
- Golden-seal

Do not use this program if you are pregnant. See your health care professional first.

lems with other trace minerals. Whenever possible use balanced multi-mineral and vitamin supplements to ensure a balanced supply of all the associated nutrients needed for utilization of zinc.

Changing Your Diet

So, you want to change your diet for the better, but you're not sure where to begin. Dietary change need not be a frightening spectre of brown rice and bean sprouts. Nor will preparing healthy food take longer or be more expensive. Just a few simple changes will be enough to begin to improve your health, energy levels, and appearance in a matter of months.

A word of advice, though. Don't try to change all aspects of your diet overnight. Remember, you are trying to change the eating habits of a lifetime, and if you want the changes to be more than a temporary "diet," take your time. Be proud of just one small change at a time.

Developing New Shopping Habits

Change number one is made from behind the wheels of a supermarket cart. It entails refraining from filling the cart with an array of high-calorie, sugar-laden junk foods such as cookies, cakes, chocolates, candy, and sugared breakfast cereals. Beware the salty villains, too—potato chips are no substitute!

These foods are all high in saturated fat (the kind that slowly clogs up your arteries), with the exception of some breakfast cereals. They are full of empty calories—that is, calories that are accompanied by only very small amounts of nutrients. And of course continually snacking on these foods will keep your dentist (and your bathroom scales) busy!

If you're searching for substitutes, start thinking grapes, apples, carrots, homemade popcorn, unsalted nuts and seeds. . . . Wander over to the produce aisle for fresh ideas.

Out With the White and in With the Brown

Replace all your refined, denatured white grains with unrefined whole-grain products. White, marshmallowy bread can be replaced with delicious (and infinitely more satisfying) whole wheat bread. Gluey white rice can be replaced with brown rice, with its appealing nutty taste and vastly superior nutritional content. Try whole wheat pasta instead of white. Switching to unrefined grains is an easy way to increase the fiber content of your diet, and in so doing to decrease your likelihood of developing bowel cancer, heart disease, and blood sugar disorders such as diabetes or hypoglycemia. Unrefined grains also provide you with much greater supplies of vitamins and minerals. Refining grains destroys large amounts of useful B complex vitamins and vitamin E in particular.

Choosing a Good Bread

People who consume high-fiber diets rarely suffer from chronic constipation. Be aware that a lot of brown or supposedly "whole grain" breads are really just white breads with a small amount of whole wheat flour added for coloring purposes. Breads that are made from "wheaten flour" are made from white flour! When choosing a whole grain bread, do the "brick" test. If it feels like a brick (and not a bag of cottonwool) it is probably whole grain. Confirm this by reading labels. Ingredients are listed with the greatest quantity ingredients first. If the label lists wheaten flour (meaning white flour), and then whole grain flour, it falls into the cottonwool bread family.

More Fruits and Vegetables

Increase your intake of fresh fruits and vegetables. Naturopaths have been singing the virtues of fruits and vegetables for hundreds of years, but it is only relatively recently that modern scientific research has confirmed what the naturopaths have intuitively known for centuries. Eating large amounts of fruits and vegetables protects you from a whole array of diseases such as diabetes, bowel cancer and all other cancers, obesity, and constipation.

FOOD SOURCES OF VITAMINS AND MINERALS

- Vitamin A (Retinol) — Liver, fish liver oils, egg yolk, dairy products

- Beta-carotene — Leafy green vegetables, yellow- and orange-colored fruits and vegetables

- Vitamin B_1 (Thiamine) — Wheat germ, bran, whole wheat flour, brown rice, brewer's yeast, blackstrap molasses, sunflower seeds, peanuts, avocado

- Vitamin B_2 (Riboflavin) — Brewer's yeast, organ meats, oily fish (herring, mackerel, trout), dark green vegetables, nori seaweed

- Vitamin B_3 (Niacin) — Liver and organ meats, poultry, fish, peanuts, yeast, wheat germ, avocado, dates

- Vitamin B_5 (Pantothenic acid) — Organ meats, brewer's yeast, fish, chicken, peanuts, whole grain cereals, peas, cauliflower, avocado

- Vitamin B_6 (Pyridoxine) — Organ meats, wheat germ, egg yolk, soybeans, peanuts, walnuts, bananas, prunes, cauliflower, cabbage, avocado

- Vitamin B_9 (Folacin) — Green leafy vegetables, beets, asparagus, broccoli, liver, kidney, oranges, pineapples, bananas, berries, brewer's yeast

- Vitamin B_{12} (Cobalamin) — Meat, most fish, crabs, oysters, egg yolk, milk, yogurt

- Biotin — Egg yolk, liver, brewer's yeast, brown rice, nuts, milk

- Choline — Soybeans, egg yolk, brewer's yeast, wheat germ, fish, peanuts, leafy green vegetables, organ meats

- Inositol — Whole grains, oranges, molasses, liver, brewer's yeast

- PABA (Para-amino-benzoic acid) — Liver, brewer's yeast, wheat germ, rice, eggs, molasses

- Vitamin C (Ascorbic acid) — Citrus fruits, rosehips, acerola cherries, melons, strawberries, broccoli, brussel sprouts, tomatoes, cabbage, peppers

• Vitamin D (Calciferol)	Fish liver oils, egg yolk, butter, liver
• Vitamin E (Tocopherol)	Vegetable oils (especially wheat germ oil), seed and nut oils, wheat germ, nuts and seeds
• Vitamin F (Essential fatty acids)	Dark green leafy vegetables, most green plants, alfalfa, kelp, blackstrap molasses, polyunsaturated oils such as safflower, liver, milk, egg yolk, fish liver oils
• Calcium	Green leafy vegetables, broccoli, cauliflower, peas, beans, nuts, molasses, sesame seeds, soybeans, dairy products
• Chromium	Brewer's yeast, beef, liver, whole wheat, oysters, potatoes, wheat germ, beets, mushrooms
• Iodine	Fish, shellfish, sea vegetables, kelp, vegetables grown in iodine-rich soil
• Iron	Wheat germ, beef, liver, pork, lamb, chicken, shellfish, clams, oysters, egg yolk, millet, oats, brown rice, dried peas and beans, nuts and seeds, green leafy vegetables, dried fruit, yellow fruits
• Magnesium	Dark green leafy vegetables, nuts, seeds, legumes, brown rice, soybeans, tofu, whole grains, wheat germ, millet
• Phosphorus	Protein foods (meat and fish), sugar, soft drinks
• Potassium	Spinach, parsley, lettuce, broccoli, peas, tomatoes, potatoes (especially the skins), oranges, bananas, apples, avocados, wheat germ, nuts, seeds
• Selenium	Brewer's yeast, wheat germ, liver, butter, fish, lamb, Brazil-nuts, barley, oats, brown rice, shellfish, garlic, onions, mushrooms
• Sodium	Seafood, beef, celery, beets, carrots, artichokes, sodium chloride (salt) in most processed foods
• Zinc	Oysters, red meat, herring, egg yolk, chicken, whole wheat, rye and oats, pecan nuts, Brazil-nuts, pumpkin seeds

Green, yellow, and orange vegetables contain large amounts of beta-carotene, the vegetable form of vitamin A. Science has proven that this vitamin is a cell-protecting anti-oxidant (like vitamins E and C), and helps to prevent cells from mutating into dangerous cancers.

Fiber—Facts and Fallacies

Fiber is the part of food which is not digested by your body, but instead is passed out virtually unchanged in your stool. Dietary fiber comes from fruits and vegetables, unrefined grains, and beans and legumes. Those good old traditional staples of meat and dairy products do not contain any fiber, only large dollops of calories and fats. Most Americans don't get enough fiber in their diet, and pay the penalty with any number of gastrointestinal disorders ranging from chronic constipation and hemorrhoids to bowel cancer and a frighteningly high incidence of cardiovascular disease. Yes, heart disease and fiber intake seem to be linked.

Those countries with the highest fiber intake also have the lowest incidence of heart disease. Certain types of fiber such as pectin and gum help lower blood cholesterol levels. Those fibers are contained in citrus fruits, apples and pears, and oats and legumes such as beans, chickpeas, peas, and lentils.

Fiber foods provide lots of appetite-satisfying bulk without supplying huge amounts of calories. Consequently, eating a high-fiber diet is

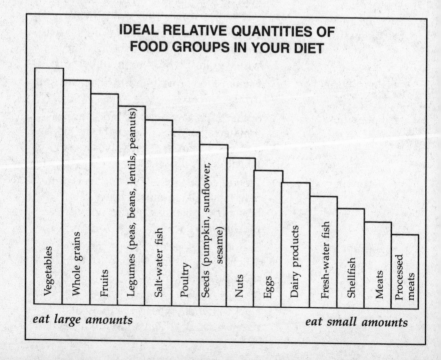

usually kind to your waistline as well as your heart and your stomach! Instead of adding an obligatory tablespoon of unappetizing bran to your refined breakfast cereals, look at more appetizing and effective ways of increasing your fiber intake.

Switch to a true whole grain bread to increase your daily fiber intake dramatically. Grains lose most of their fiber content when they are refined. Use brown rice instead of white, and substitute whole grain pasta for the white variety. Add liberal quantities of fresh fruit and vegetables, and you can be fairly sure of reaching your recommended daily fiber intake of 30 g without having to resort to dry bran flakes! (Then again, if you're one of those folks who loves cold bran cereal, stick with it.)

On the Subject of Fat

Some easy ways to reduce your fat intake:

- Use low-fat dairy products such as skim milk, low- or non-fat cottage cheese, low-fat yogurts, and low-fat hard cheeses such as Edam and Alpine Lace.
- Cut down your red meat intake and use more chicken, fish, and vegetarian proteins instead.
- Steam, grill, or dry-roast foods instead of frying or oil-roasting.
- Be aware of less apparent sources of dietary fats such as potato chips, tacos, roasted peanuts, chocolate, cakes, cookies, and crackers.

AMERICAN DIET

Too much	*Not enough*
• Calories	• Fiber
• Fat	• Fresh fruits and vegetables
• Saturated fat	• Nutrients including: calcium, magnesium, zinc, selenium, iron, B vitamins, vitamin E, essential fatty acids
• Hydrogenated oil	
• Protein	
• Salt	
• Sugar	
• Alcohol	
• Dairy products	
• Red meat	
• Phosphorus	

- If you eat peanut butter, look for the jars with a thick layer of oil swimming on top. They may look unappealing, but they are far better for you. Most commercial peanut butters today have been hydrogenated to stop the peanut paste separating from the oil. In doing so, the peanut butter is transformed into a saturated (and potentially unhealthy) fat.
- Pay a bit extra and buy cold-pressed oils in preference to the chemically extracted commercial oils. Always buy cold-pressed oils packed in dark glass bottles, as this greatly reduces the likelihood of purchasing a rancid oil. Store oil in the fridge always. Never use any oil for more than one cooking, and never allow the oil to heat to temperatures causing it to smoke. Excessive heating alters the structure of the oil, causing the formation of carcinogenic chemicals.

Drinks Count, Too

Have a look at what you drink. Do you reach for a caffeine fix every hour or so? If coffee and tea drinking is more than an occasional pleasure, you could experiment with some caffeine-free alternatives. Try some of the wide range of herbal teas available. They don't all look and taste like pond weed. Pleasant and health-giving teas include rosehip (rich in vitamin C and iron); peppermint (especially good for strengthening the stomach and improving digestion); and chamomile (a calming and sedative tea just right for a nightcap). The fruity range of herbal teas is delicious and a tasty introduction. Why not try replacing some of your coffee with almond or ginger tea, a cereal coffee, dandelion coffee, or carob drink?

If you just can't live without that coffee taste, you could alternate between cereal coffees and decaffeinated coffee, but make sure that your coffee is decaffeinated through a water process, not a chemical process. There is evidence linking the chemical process to cancer.

A Little More on the Subject of Caffeine

Caffeine is one of those ubiquitous drugs that many people partake of as and when they feel like it. In fact, sharing a cup of coffee with friends is one of the foremost social rituals. It is strange that this substance can make its way into your life without demanding a second thought. In fact, it is known to produce a wide variety of unpleasant physiological changes when taken in large amounts. Caffeine pops up in more places than the coffee pot—tea, cola drinks, chocolate, medications such as "stay awake" pills and asthma drugs, all supply more caffeine.

Caffeine stimulates your central nervous system, with as little as one cup of freshly brewed coffee producing a noticeable "pep up" effect as it clears your thinking and boosts your energy. Along with these seemingly beneficial effects come less obvious, and detrimental, effects on your cardiovascular system, including raising your blood pressure and speeding your heart rate. Caffeine leads to many of the symptoms of anxiety and panic attacks. Caffeine is also a mild laxative and a diuretic, increasing the loss of your water-soluble vitamins in your urine.

As is the case with any drug, the more often you use caffeine, the more you need to get the "high." Over time you can become addicted to caffeine, needing it to function normally, and exhibiting proper withdrawal symptoms if you fail to get it. You can consider yourself a high user of caffeine if your intake is 500 mg or more a day. This is the equivalent of about four cups of drip-percolated coffee, or about seven cups of instant coffee (remember to take into account all the other less obvious caffeine sources). If this is you, you should be aware of the indisputable scientific evidence of undesirable side-effects of use at these levels.

Besides revving up your nervous system to hyperactive levels, resulting in irritability, nervousness, and panic attacks, coffee can also irritate your gastrointestinal system by increasing the acid production in your stomach—obviously not a good idea if you are prone to ulcers or acid reflux. By making you run to the bathroom frequently, coffee increases the loss of a number of vital water-soluble nutrients, including the B complex, vitamin C, potassium, magnesium, and zinc. It also reduces your absorption of iron and calcium, especially if you drink it within an hour of a meal.

All these effects may be considered fairly minor compared with the harm caffeine can do to your cardiovascular system. By raising your blood pressure, it increases your risk of developing clogging of the arteries and heart disease. It also changes your blood fats composition, increasing blood cholesterol and triglyceride levels. By stimulating overproduction of an adrenal hormone called norepinephrine, caffeine also causes your blood vessels to constrict, making it harder for your heart to pump the blood around your body.

If you suffer from fibrocystic breast disease (see A-Z), you really should stay away from coffee completely. There is a large body of research linking this problem with excessive caffeine use, and certainly women who stop using this drug often find a dramatic reduction in the severity of their breast problems. Other women's problems associated with high caffeine intake include an association with ovarian cancer, and a higher incidence of birth defects and spontaneous abortions when used during pregnancy.

If you drink five or six cups a day, you may now decide to come off coffee. But be prepared for some rather unpleasant withdrawal effects. Most commonly you will start with a thumping headache within about 12 hours of your last cup. You may experience nervous system symptoms such as irritability, depression, insomnia, nervousness, and shaking. But hang in there and persevere and your symptoms will soon pass.

As is the case with kicking the nicotine habit, you will find the job easier if you pay some attention to your diet and nutrient intake at the same time. Consuming a mainly alkaline reaction diet (see nicotine detoxification, p. 96), along with a high intake of water, will help reduce withdrawal symptoms. Boost your vitamin C reserves with frequent doses of calcium ascorbate, and use a high potency stress B complex two or three times a day. Gradually tapering off your caffeine intake over a week or two seems to be a lot less traumatic than going cold turkey. You can try using grain or dandelion coffees in place of the real thing, and experiment with some of the "pep up" herbal teas such as peppermint, ginseng, and ginger tea.

Weight-Reducing Diets

No look at diet and nutrition would be complete without considering the subject of weight-loss diets—a subject that many Western women are sadly preoccupied with, often with dire consequences that include a horrifyingly high incidence of eating illnesses such as anorexia and bulimia. Fashion magazines and TV ads contribute to the obsession with endless "before" pictures of seemingly miserable and overweight people transformed into beautiful and happy "afters."

While it's true that losing weight has something to do with what you put in your mouth, in reality it is a lot more complex. Being significantly overweight will predispose you to a range of debilitating and deadly health problems including diabetes, heart disease, high blood pressure, kidney disease, varicose veins, and gallbladder problems, to name a few. If you are truly overweight, you are running a risk of future health problems, which can be greatly minimized by shedding your excess now.

However, many women in America go on one diet after another, when they are not really overweight to begin with. More often than not, an exercise program designed to tone and strengthen muscles will produce more improvement than any diet.

What Happens to Your Body When You Diet

People become fat in the first place when they take in more energy (calories) than they use in a day's activity. The surplus calories are then transformed into fat and laid away as a safety store for the next time they control a famine. Fortunately, though, famine never comes, and those little fat stores grow and grow.

Each person has a unique basal metabolic rate (BMR), influenced by size, age, nutritional status, and genes. The BMR is a measure of the amount of energy your body requires to perform the simple staying alive functions of maintaining normal body temperature and muscle tone and keeping all the vital organs functioning.

Have you ever marveled (with a hint of green in your eye) how your skinny friend can gorge herself from dawn to dusk, and still fit into her size 10 jeans? Part of the reason may be her high metabolic rate. Her body uses up a huge amount of energy simply performing the "staying alive" functions, leaving little surplus to be converted into fat. And yes, genes do have something to do with her luck, but you don't have to resign yourself to accepting your genetic legacy of being overweight. It is now proven and widely acknowledged that you can change your own BMR for the better! Although children of these parents often have lower BMRs than children of slim parents, their BMR can be greatly increased through following a specific type of exercise regime. BMR is also affected by your ratio of muscle to fat. The greater your percentage of muscle, the greater your metabolic rate. This is one of the long-term beneficial effects that regular exercise has on your weight.

How Dieting Can Result in Weight Gain

Is your diet as full of nutrients as it should be? Prolonged under-nutrition *slows down* the BMR, making you more likely to gain weight when you overindulge in the pleasures of eating.

Ironically, the single factor that adversely affects your BMR more than any other is *dieting*! In its infinite wisdom, the body interprets a diet as being a famine, and a threat to its survival. It automatically drastically reduces the number of calories it uses for its basic organic maintenance functions. As these functions account for about 65 percent of the energy used by your body, this can seriously affect your weight loss attempts. For example, a 160-pound person uses about 70 calories an hour while sleeping. This drops dramatically to 40 calories an hour when he or she is dieting.

Your body also becomes more efficient at storing fat with repeated dieting. When you take in any kind of dietary fat, your body releases a digestive enzyme called lipase to break it down before it enters your intestines. This enables your body to use or store the fat more easily. In chronic dieters, this enzyme becomes more active, facilitating the storage of fat in the body. Within two days of beginning a very strict diet, your metabolic rate slows by about 15 percent, your energy requirements drop, and the storage of "excess" energy becomes much more efficient.

Strict dieting prepares your body for a more efficient storage of calories. A recent UCLA study found that people following 1000-calorie-a-day diets showed a reduction in BMR of up to 40 percent within a matter of days of commencing the diet. They calculated that this alone would account for a weight *gain* of 28 pounds in one year.

The Set Point Theory

Basal metabolic rate may partially explain your skinny friend, but she may also be the fortunate victim of her body's own "set point." The "set point" theory proposes that each person has a natural biological weight compatible with his or her metabolism. That is, you have a kind of fat thermostat which seeks to maintain a constant amount of fat in the body. Experiments carried out during the Second World War, using conscientious objectors, illustrate how fighting individual set point, through constant dieting, is both destructive and futile. These men lost weight when placed on a strictly limited calorie intake. However, as soon as they came off the enforced starvation, they ate ravenously with appetites that could not be satiated until they reached their original weight and muscle/fat ratio. Once they reached their ideal weight it fluctuated by only 3 or so pounds a month, no matter how much they ate.

An opposite but equally illuminating experiment again supported the "set point" theory. This time prisoners were encouraged to overeat to try to increase their body weight by 20 percent. Only two of the 20 volunteers managed to achieve this, despite adding up to 2030 calories to their daily diet. As soon as the experiment finished, all the men found they ate less than half the amount of their original daily diets, and exercised through choice, rapidly dropping to their starting weight.

Both experiments prove that the body does its utmost to maintain the particular amount of fat it requires by altering appetite, the desire for physical activity, and the metabolic rate. People who have been fat from childhood are likely to have naturally high set points, while those who begin regular physical exercise while young are likely to have low set points. Some people will never be able to emulate the socially desirable reed thinness of the ideal of Western physical perfection—one version of the ideal, that is. They will simply make themselves miserable, frustrated, and quite possibly fatter, in their futile quest for thinness.

Any "professional" dieter will attest to the amazing weight loss/gain yo-yo that frequent dieting can cause. First you lose your weight (and simultaneously depress your metabolic rate—allowing your body to maintain its normal activity on fewer and fewer calories) and treat yourself to that new dress. Then you start eating what you consider to be a sensible maintenance diet, only to find the scales steadily creeping back up to your original weight! Your body has adapted itself to self-preservation on a meager diet, and now what was once a maintenance diet is a fattening diet.

As well as resulting in a frustrating inability to lose weight and maintain your loss, yo-yo dieting can have other more serious consequences. For example, women who live on one diet after another often cause their body fat stores to redistribute from their thighs and hips (where women are supposed to have more fat), to their abdomens. Excess weight carried above the waist has been shown to increase greatly your chances of developing diabetes and heart disease. All the research now shows that cycles of weight loss and gain do indeed increase your heart attack risk. A major study monitoring more than 5000 people for 40 years found that people who gained 10 percent more weight increased their risk of heart disease by 30 percent. When they lost 10 percent of their weight they only decreased their heart attack risk by 20 percent, thus resulting in a 10 percent net increase in risk every time they went through the loss/gain yo-yo.

Tied in with the set point theory is the fat cell theory. At certain times of your life (before birth, during your infancy, and then again in adolescence) your body creates new fat cells. The number produced depends upon a number of factors including genetics, and also the amount of food you consume at these three crucial stages. The more food you eat, the more fat cells are produced. During your adult years, instead of producing new fat cells, you simply increase the size of your existing fat cells, in response to your food intake. Whenever you eat more calories than you actually use, your fat cells swell in size. People who stay slim despite eating large amounts most probably have a smaller number of fat cells than those individuals who gain weight by simply looking at a cream cake. They also tend to have faster metabolisms and a lower set point.

Exercise and Your Metabolism

So what is the missing link in all this depressing talk of metabolism? It is *exercise*. Even a moderate amount of exercise can help speed up your metabolic rate, lower your set point, and decrease your appetite. Twenty minutes of aerobic exercise each day is enough to boost your metabolic rate for the next 15 hours. Cycling, brisk walking, aerobics, or swimming for 20 to 30 minutes each day will make your diet a healthier and far more effective mission, as your body maintains (or even increases) its BMR and continues to use a high number of calories for basic "staying alive" purposes.

By the way, 20 minutes is the absolute minimum amount of continuous exercise required to kick start your metabolic rate. Increase your exercise session to 30 to 45 minutes and you boost your BMR for a whole 24 hours.

Of course, this level of exercise is a goal, not a starting point. Just as changing your shopping and your eating habits works best in gradual stages, you'll want to make a few changes in the right direction to get yourself started. *Any* exercise is better than none at all. The next chapter will guide you through the basics of setting up an exercise program ideally suited to your tastes and needs. You may surprise yourself and find you *enjoy* getting into better shape.

Exercise also makes it easier to overcome those excruciating sugar cravings that seem to go hand in hand with any serious dieting. Exercise stabilizes your blood sugar level—lowering it if it is too high, or increasing it if it is too low (as is often the case with dieting). Instead of battling with your willpower at the cupboard door, try a 10-minute jog, or a brisk walk, or a bounce on a mini-trampoline. When you've finished, the craving will probably have disappeared.

When You Eat Makes a Difference

Did you know that it's not just what you eat that affects your weight, but also when you eat? Any dieter who virtually starves all day and then eats a large meal at night is taking two steps down for one step up. All day long their body receives the message of "red alert—famine conditions." It responds by drastically lowering the metabolic rate. Then comes evening, along with a reasonable input of calories. However, instead of burning them up in the process of body maintenance, the famine-activated body simply turns these calories to *fat*.

American nutritionist Ronald Gatty recently provided indisputable proof that timing makes a difference in dieting. In an experiment, one group of subjects took the bulk of their food in the mornings, while the other group did the opposite, taking most of their food in the latter part of the day. Besides this one restriction, both groups ate whatever they wanted. Yes, you've guessed—the group eating late in the day gained about half a pound per week. On the other hand, the early eaters actually lost weight at the rate of about two and three-quarter pounds per week.

A similar experiment was performed, but with both groups eating the same total number of calories in a day. Again, the early eaters lost weight while the late eaters gained. Common sense tells you part of the reason why eating large amounts in the evening can be fattening. Flopping onto the sofa for several hours of television, and then into bed for the night, gives little opportunity for calories to be burned through physical activity.

There are other more complicated reasons for this phenomenon, to do with biochemical and hormonal fluctuations through the day. Whenever you eat, your pancreas releases the hormone insulin, which is responsible for controlling blood sugar levels and for taking excess sugar out of the blood, to be stored. Early in the day insulin levels are lower, and consequently less fat can be stored at this time, and more calories are made available to be burned during activity. Late in the day, insulin levels are higher, making fat storage easier and more likely!

There are a host of other hormones (such as adrenalin, glucagon, cortisol, and testosterone) that have similar time-related fluctuations, making digestion and energy use more efficient early in the day.

So now you may see how timing of meals and regular exercise can help you lose or maintain body weight, before you even count a single calorie. You may well be able to lose your excess pounds by simply eating the bulk of your total food intake before 1 p.m., and gradually increasing your aerobic exercise to 30 minutes or more each day. In the long term, these simple lifestyle changes will be more effective than falling into the psychological trap of going on a diet, with all its connotations of deprivation and, often, failure.

Counting Calories Is Only Part of the Picture

The diets of the future may not even mention the word calorie. More and more research indicates that counting calories is only a small part of the weight-loss picture. It is not just the quantity, but the quality of your food that affects your weight. Bodies react differently to calories supplied from different types of foods. For example, energy supplied by fats and simple (refined) carbohydrates are processed differently then those supplied by complex (unrefined) carbohydrates. Almost 100 percent of the calories supplied by fats are converted into fat on your body. Conversely, only a tiny percentage of energy supplied by complex carbohydrates and protein is converted into body fat.

Considering the average American diet, it is hardly surprising that weight loss is a mega-dollar industry here. Typical diets abound with saturated fats in the form of red meat, butter, cheese, whole milk, potato chips, fried foods, cakes, cookies, chocolate, and the list goes on and on! (See the chart on p. 63.) The average American obtains between 37 and 42 percent of total calories from fats. Most nutrition experts agree that you need to cut this fat down to 20 to 30 percent of total calorie intake to optimize your weight loss and then maintain this loss.

Another main source of calories is simple carbohydrates—foods that are high in sugars and white flour products. These refined carbohydrates are metabolized differently than the complex carbohydrates supplied by whole grains, fruits, and vegetables. Simple carbohydrates flood your bloodstream with a sudden and excessive quantity of sugar. This stimulates a hair-trigger and dramatic response from the pancreas, which pours large amounts of insulin into your sugar-laden bloodstream. The insulin quickly takes the sugar from the blood into the cells, and unless burned up immediately through exercise, your chocolate brownie is rapidly converted to spare tire.

Complex carbohydrates, on the other hand, are digested slowly, releasing a gradual trickle of sugar into your bloodstream, and providing a long-lasting energy boost. Most of this sugar remains available to be burned off through exercise and general body maintenance.

The complex carbohydrates of fruit, vegetables, and whole grains aid your weight loss in other ways, too. By supplying large amounts of fiber, they satisfy your need for oral gratification (that is, they give your chewing muscles a good workout!), and they help you to feel full and satisfied for longer after a meal.

What you now know may mean an end to calorie counters, deprivation, and naked lettuce leaves—for life!

Weight-Loss Boosters

Besides adopting a sensible eating regime and increasing your energy output through regular exercise, there are certain natural substances and dietary practices that will make the process of weight loss easier and perhaps less painful.

Water is one of your best friends when you are shedding weight. As well as suppressing your appetite, drinking generous amounts of water helps your body metabolize its fat stores and ensures regular bowel movements and waste detoxification. Drinking at least eight glasses of water a day, with a generous intake half an hour before meals, is an easy and healthy way to reduce your appetite.

Liquid chlorophyll can also help reduce your food cravings. Taken in doses as small as a teaspoon added to a glass of water, twice a day, this green plant extract improves digestion and your body's utilization of ingested nutrients. When you are adequately nourished, your desire for food is lessened and following a sensible eating plan is easier.

Essential fatty acids, both in the form of supplements and naturally occurring dietary sources, will stimulate your weight loss by improving fatty acid metabolism. A cheap way of obtaining the GLA (gamma-linoleic acid) and EPA (eicosapentaenoic acid) needed is to add three or four teaspoons of cold-pressed linseed (flax) oil to your diet each day. Remember, though, that whenever you increase your intake of any type of fat (including essential fatty acids) your requirements of vitamin E also increase.

Simply using certain herb teas can benefit your weight-loss program. Parsley tea is a great source of iron, chlorophyll, and vitamin C and is also highly diuretic, increasing your urine flow and helping your body eliminate toxins released through the breakdown of fat cells. Other diuretic teas include juniper berry and rosehip. Fennel tea is appetite-reducing, or simply chewing the fennel seeds themselves provides the same effect.

Certain vitamins are particularly important at this time. B complex vitamins are vitally important for your metabolism of carbohydrates, fats, and proteins, and are especially vital for your body to burn fats for fuel.

Chapter 3

Exercise—
Keeping the Body Fit

Good health does not come with good food alone. So far you've read about nutrition and the important contribution that a healthy diet has to make in becoming and staying healthy. If you are not a particularly active person, it's tempting to think that as long as you eat well you'll stay well. It's true that eating well is part of the picture, but regular exercise is vitally important, too. It's like filling a car with premium-grade gasoline and then leaving it to set in the garage for a year. When you come to use it, you'll find all kinds of mechanical (physical) problems have developed. If you neglect to use this brilliantly designed piece of machinery called the human body, it will stiffen, injure easily, become out of condition, and it might just break down on you.

Why Is Regular Exercise Important?

Pick up any book on exercise and you'll find a dozen or more good reasons for getting up off the couch and getting moving. In particular, regular exercise provides the following benefits for your body:

- It dramatically reduces your chances of developing heart disease, high blood pressure, clogging of the arteries, angina, and heart failure. This is achieved through an increase in the size of the heart muscle along with an increase in its efficiency (that is, the amount of blood it can pump with each contraction), and a decrease in the amount of oxygen your body needs both at rest and during exercise. Regular exercise also produces changes in your blood fats or lipids, including lowering dangerous triglyceride and low-density fats, or lipids (LDLs). Even relatively small amounts of regular exercise produce a marked increase in the cardiovascular protective high-density lipids (HDLs). Studies show that jogging or walking three times a week (an average of two miles per session) increases HDLs by over 50 percent in as little as two months. It is these HDLs that help prevent the build-up of fatty plaques in your arteries (atherosclerosis), which in turn can cause high blood pressure and heart disease.

- People who exercise regularly have far fewer problems with weight gain and obesity. Regular exercisers rarely have to worry about going on a diet. This weight-regulating effect is achieved not only through the immediate short-term burning up of calories during the actual exercise, but also through a resulting sustained increase in your metabolic rate. A high metabolic rate means that you burn more calories all the time, helping to control body fat.

- Exercise helps to normalize your blood sugar levels and has a protective effect against the development of blood sugar abnormalities such as diabetes or hypoglycemia.

- Exercise is a natural tranquilizer and a great way of controlling stress levels. Aerobic exercise in particular is a great way of releasing pent-up tension, anger, and aggression. This is partly due to an increase in your body's production of natural brain opiates (tranquilizers) known as endorphins. Some frequent aerobic exercisers become addicted to these natural opiates, and suffer withdrawal symptoms of depression and irritability if they are unable to exercise!

- Regular, safe exercise maintains the health and flexibility of your joints, muscles, and tendons, as well as helping to maintain the density and strength of your bones. Strong muscles used to working, along with your increased heart strength and oxygen uptake, account for your increased levels of energy when you exercise regularly. Lounge lizards are usually also tired lizards!

- Although all these benefits of exercise apply to men, women, and children, there are some benefits that are uniquely female. Regular exercise should be an important part of your self-help regime if you suffer from PMS or period pain—it is proven to decrease the incidence and severity of these problems. Exercise during the menopausal years also reduces the incidence of many of the common menopausal complaints including depression, anxiety, hot flashes, weight gain, and osteoporosis.

Are you now convinced that getting up off the couch and putting on your walking shoes is as important as filling the fridge with vegetables and eating whole grain bread? You may agree wholeheartedly, but if you're like most people, you may also not know where to begin. That first step is always the hardest. One key to an exercise program that you'll both stick to and enjoy is selecting the right exercise for you. You need to find an activity and a schedule that fits in *realistically* with your temperament and your lifestyle. You'd be surprised how wonderful you can feel dancing or cycling, for instance, even if you can't stand jogging. Don't fight your natural inclinations (unless they're for sleeping all day!). The next section will help you zero in on just the right plan for you. A word of warning to begin with—if you have been very inactive for a long time, or if you have any medical or health problems, visit your health care practitioner before you embark on an exercise program. You need some clear guidelines as to what your personal exercise limits are.

What Kind of Exercise Is Best?

Although all exercise is of benefit to you in some way, only certain types of exercise provide all the benefits listed above—namely, aerobic exercise. Aerobic literally means "using oxygen" and that's exactly what this type of exercise makes you do. Aerobic exercise is sustained, strenuous, repetitive movement that gives your lungs and heart a real workout. Stopping-and-starting-type exercise like badminton, tennis, golf, and bowling are not aerobic (although they are still of great value to your health if those are the sports you enjoy).

True aerobic exercise includes swimming, brisk walking, jogging, cycling, and aerobic dance workouts. Because this type of exercise places a burden on your heart and lungs, it's most important that you build up to it gradually. Don't aim to go from slothdom to running three miles within the space of a few days. Not only is this guaranteed to put you off exercise for a very long time, but it can be dangerous as well. Taking your pulse regularly during exercise will help you determine how much stress you are placing on your body, and whether you should cut back, or increase your exercise intensity.

To work out what your pulse rate should be while you exercise, subtract your age from 220, and then multiply by 0.75 (a calculator may come in handy!). For example, if you are 40, your heartbeat should rise no higher than 135 beats per minute when you are exercising. When you take your pulse you don't need to take a full one-minute reading—simply count your heartbeat for 10 seconds and then multiply it by 6 to give you your rate per minute.

If you want to increase your energy levels, strengthen your heart and lungs, and boost your metabolic rate, then aerobic exercise is for you. In order to reap these rewards you need to exercise aerobically for at least 20 minutes (but preferably 30 to 45), a minimum of three times a week. Aim to make your exercise sessions as enjoyable as possible—a pleasure rather than another chore to be endured.

Whatever type of exercise you decide to embark on, there are some general practices that should be adhered to. These include religiously making time for a pre-exercise stretch and warm-up routine, and a post-exercise cool-down period (allowing ten minutes for each). Many an injury could have been prevented if only these exercise basics had not been overlooked. While all types of exercise are theoretically good for you, some also carry an element of risk, while other forms are more appropriate for certain types of people and to achieve more specific benefits.

Walking

Brisk walking is a great way to start, as it requires no special equipment, financial investment, or skill—simply a pair of sturdy, flat-soled shoes and some sunshine! Walking is also an extremely low-risk exercise, with no threat of injury short of falling off the sidewalk and twisting an ankle!

Start by walking a moderate distance, such as half a mile. Time your achievement and then gradually increase your speed and your distance over the next few weeks. Simply increasing your walking time by an extra five minutes every three days will see you safely on to a beneficial exercise program in no time. Just be careful not to settle into a stroll. Check your heart rate to see when you need to add jaunt to your step.

Jogging

If you want to move on from your walking regime when you gain in physical fitness, you may wish to choose jogging. If so, it is important that you invest in a good quality pair of running shoes, as the incidence of injury with this exercise can be quite high. Shin splints, torn or strained muscles, knee injury, or twisted ankles can all be problems if you fail to warm up properly, or if you push yourself too hard. Wearing good running shoes reduces your likelihood of injury. Whenever possible jog on soft surfaces like grass, dirt trails, or the beach. Pounding out huge distances on asphalt is a recipe for injury in the long run.

Swimming

One of the all-time top exercises, swimming works just about every one of the 500 or so muscles in your body. It's great for anyone who has a back injury or leg problems, and it is particularly good for pregnant women, as the water makes exercising easier by supporting your increased size and weight. It is not so good if you suffer from sinus problems or ear infections (unless you swim in salt water, in which case the water rushing up your nose can actually improve your sinus trouble).

Cycling

This is another great aerobic exercise, which provides a particularly good workout for the legs, but not much for the upper body. You need to be able to afford a bicycle and a helmet (a safety necessity on today's crazy roads).

Exercise and Women

No matter what your age, condition, or state of fitness, exercise is an important part of your self-help health care. You can exercise throughout pregnancy, during the postnatal period, throughout your menopausal years, and at any other stage of your life cycle. Regular exercise has been shown to help balance your hormones; decrease severity of PMS, anxiety, and depression; relieve period pain; decrease or eliminate many of the common minor health problems of pregnancy, including constipation, varicose veins, hemorrhoids, excessive weight gain, and backache; and prevent the chronic bone degeneration of osteoporosis.

So, what are you waiting for? If you are playing a vigorous sport like tennis or raquetball, or jogging, invest in a good quality sports bra, designed to provide additional breast support. This will prevent sagging or stretching of the breast tissue during exercise. Cotton underpants are also a good idea to help prevent any proliferation of vaginal yeast if you are prone to thrush, as the increased temperatures generated by exercise can provide a hospitable environment for these little nuisances to thrive.

Pregnancy and Fitness

The era of being cosseted and fussed over by concerned husbands and parents during your pregnancy has gone. Those days of strict instructions to "rest and take it easy" have been replaced with a general acknowledgment that exercising during pregnancy is as important (and in some ways more important) than at any other time of your life.

Women who exercise regularly during pregnancy have easier births, with fewer complications and shorter labors. The incidence of problems during the actual pregnancy, in particular toxemia, is also considerably lower for fit women. While pregnancy is a perfectly normal and healthy state, there are considerable extra demands placed upon your body—demands that will be all the more readily met by a fit and supple body. Even in a totally normal pregnancy you will experience considerable weight gain, which itself causes strain on your back (especially your lower back) and your abdomen. The volume of blood coursing through your body is also greatly increased, causing your heart to work harder all the time. And when it comes to the actual birth, there will be some real "labor" to do, akin to running a marathon in some cases!

You may be wondering what kind of exercise you can do while you're pregnant. The answer is virtually anything, except contact sports, in which you place yourself in danger of being knocked over or knocked in the abdomen. Don't take up any new strenuous sport during your pregnancy. If you were accustomed to running several miles a day before you became pregnant, it's okay to continue running for as long as you feel comfortable (providing your pregnancy is completely normal and healthy). It is not a good idea, however, to embark suddenly on a jogging regime during your pregnancy if you have rarely had a pair of running shoes on your feet before. If you want to start an exercise program, by all means start regular brisk walking or swimming, but not jogging. If you live near a swimming pool, check if they offer water aerobic classes, as these are a great form of safe aerobic exercise, especially useful for pregnant women. When you attend an pre-natal clinic, you can ask for a list of exercises specifically designed to meet your special requirements during pregnancy, and as preparation for the birth.

There are a number of "don'ts" to heed when you start your pregnancy exercise program. These include:

- Avoid getting excessively overheated during your exercising, as your increased temperature can cause harm to your developing baby. Never perform any aerobic exercise to the point where you are unable to talk comfortably while exercising. If you can't do this, then you are placing an excessively great load on your cardiovascular system.
- Avoid any type of exercise that places great strain on your lower back, or overstretches your abdominal muscles. For example, don't do sit-ups with your legs straight out in front of you. Always do sit-ups with your knees bent and the soles of your feet kept flat on the floor.
- In the latter months of pregnancy, avoid exercises that involve lying on your stomach or flat on your back.

You should also have specific aims when designing your pregnancy exercise routine:

- Design a program that involves aerobic activity to increase your fitness levels, oxygen uptake, and strength of your heart; and also include stretching exercises to increase your suppleness and lessen the likelihood of pregnancy backache, as well as preparing you for birth.
- Begin every session with 10 minutes of warm-up exercises to stretch muscles, tendons, and ligaments and warm your muscles. This should always be a part of every exercise session, but it is especially important during pregnancy, when rising hormone levels cause a softening of your connective tissue and ligaments, making you especially prone to injury.
- End each session with a cool-down rather than abruptly stopping your activity. This too will decrease the incidence of injury.

Don't Forget Your Pelvic Floor!

Pelvic floor exercises are probably the most important exercise you can perform during your pregnancy, and then forevermore. They provide a work-out to that sheath of muscle underneath all your lower abdominal organs (in particular your bladder and uterus), and give the support that keeps them securely where they belong. When these rarely used muscles weaken, you can end up with prolapses of the bladder and uterus (both of which are extremely common and responsible for many of the surgical admissions to gynecological wards).

Weak pelvic floor muscles also account for the annoying bladder incontinence that often occurs after you have had a baby. If you avoid the jumping exercises at the gym because you can't control your bladder, then you need to start doing pelvic floor exercises—*today*!

The specific exercises designed to strengthen and tone these muscles are named after a Los Angeles surgeon by the name of Kegel. Before you can begin to perform the exercises, you have to find your pelvic floor muscles. The easiest time to do this is probably when you are urinating. Next time you pass water, try to tighten your muscles to stop the flow of urine. The muscles you use to achieve this are your pelvic floor muscles. (By the way, if you fail to stop the urine flow, it's another indication that you need to perform these exercises regularly.)

So now that you know where the muscles are, how do you do the exercises? Imagine that your pelvic floor is like an elevator in a tall building. Start with the elevator at the bottom floor (pelvic floor totally relaxed) and then gradually draw the elevator up through the building by gradually tightening the pelvic floor muscles. Move the elevator slowly, floor by floor, by increasing the muscle contraction gradually. Between each increase, hold the current contraction for five seconds before increasing it to the next "floor," where you hold it for another five seconds.

Once your muscles are as tight as they can go, repeat the procedure in reverse, gradually relaxing your muscles, floor by floor, until they are completely relaxed again. Try to repeat these exercises in sets of five, with about 10 repetitions a day (making a total of 50 times a day). Remember that there's really no excuse for not performing these "private exercises" because they can be done anywhere at any time—while you're driving the car, sitting at your desk, or watching television.

Exercise and Your Back

Back problems account for a huge number of missed working days. If you have a history of back problems, you can greatly help yourself by embarking on an ongoing "back-safe" exercise regime. By working on increasing your spine flexibility and strengthening your abdominal muscles (so important to guard against lower back problems), you will quickly see an improvement in your comfortable range of movement, and a decrease in your incidence of acute back pain.

Walking, cycling, and swimming (especially) are all safe aerobic options for you if you suffer from back problems. Jogging is not advisable, as the lower back takes quite a pounding when you run. There are other forms of exercise that many back sufferers swear by. These include yoga, simple stretching exercises, and tai chi.

A Back-to-Basics Look at Back Care

It's the end of a typical day of living. You've heaved bags of shopping, hauled your toddler in and out of the car, done some gardening, and been for a jog. And now . . . your back is killing you! It may be a small comfort to know that you are far from alone in your suffering. Back pain is a modern-day scourge.

An American study at the National Centre for Health Statistics shows that severe, long-term back pain causes more visits to American doctors than any other problem, with at least two million new cases each year. Back injury and pain are hazards of living for everyone, but women have some additional high-risk factors. Pregnancy, with its dramatic and rapid figure-altering effects, is one of them. The rigors of the birth itself can cause back trauma, which can be the launch of a lifetime of suffering, if not treated properly. And the bone-thinning disease osteoporosis mostly strikes women, and greatly weakens the bones by leaching their calcium away.

As if that isn't enough, many women add to their spinal problems in the name of fashion and beauty. High heels have a disastrous effect on the natural alignment of the spine. By tilting the hips forward, high heels abnormally exaggerate the curve at the bottom of your spine. This may look attractive to some, but its price is often a legacy of back pain.

The human spine is an exquisitely designed piece of mechanical engineering which enables you to live an evolutionarily unique existence as a two-legged, upright animal. The spine is made up of three stacked curves: the neck (cervical), rib cage (thoracic), and lower back (lumbar). These curves give you a balanced center of gravity and allow to walk along a windy street without being blown over. Your body is designed so that a healthy posture leaves all your vertebrae and back muscles in a comfortable state of equalibrium. That is a condition of relaxation, where the vertebrae float freely upon each other with no strain. Sadly, human spines were not designed with modern living in mind. Combine poor posture, badly designed furniture, saggy mattresses, high heels, and bulging midriffs and you have a spinal time bomb just waiting to explode.

Through years of unwitting back abuse the curves in your spine change, usually becoming more exaggerated. The muscles in your back are forced to shorten or lengthen to cope with the abnormal curves. Your new center of gravity causes some of your back muscles to stay permanently contracted and tensed. As the months and years pass, these contracted muscles become hardened, ropy, and inflexible. Tight muscles alone can be enough to cause back pain, and a rigid back is an intolerant back. Simply stooping to pick up a paper clip from the floor may be the final straw that leaves you squirming in agony and rushing to the osteopath's clinic.

How Can You Prevent Back Problems?

Common sense tells you that *prevention* is the cheapest and least painful solution to back problems, but where do you start? Beginning with the fuel you run on, your bones and muscles can only be as healthy as the raw materials you provide for them. A healthy spine begins at the dinner table (and remember not to slouch!). A range of vitamins and minerals are essential for spinal health, in particular vitamins C, E, and D, the minerals calcium and magnesium, and adequate protein. Collagen is a protein substance that makes up tendons, bones, and cartilages, which give the body support and strength. Vitamin C is one of the main building blocks of this collagen, and healthy collagen means a healthier back.

Dr. Greenwood, an American professor of neurosurgery, has performed dozens of experiments that prove the value of vitamin C supplements for back problems. He found that patients with spinal disc problems could often avoid surgery simply by taking vitamin C supplements! Today, Dr. Greenwood starts all his back patients on 1500 mg of vitamin C daily, and in doing so has dramatically reduced his surgery list. (Refer to the previous chapter for more about vitamin C.)

Ninety-eight percent of your body's calcium is stored in your bones. This calcium is the most important (but not the only) mineral for the formation of the body's rigid structural support system. A lack of dietary calcium is one of the main factors implicated in the development of the bone-thinning disease osteoporosis (see A-Z for more detail).

Other changes, apart from diet, can also help to safeguard your back. If back pain is a real problem for you and you are overweight, give some serious thought to a weight-reducing diet. An overweight body places constant, excessive stress on your spine. A flabby and voluminous abdomen strains the lower back and makes it curve excessively inward, causing pain. Pregnant women often suffer terribly from backache toward the end of pregnancy. Extra weight, changed posture, and ligament-softening hormones are the cause of this suffering.

The importance of toned abdominal muscles cannot be overstated when it comes to preventing lower back problems. Weak abdominals cause postural compensation, with a shift of your weight to the back. This causes your pelvis to tilt forward and your hips to stick out correspondingly to the rear. This places a great strain on your lower back muscles and vertebrae. It doesn't take long for these lower back muscles to start aching.

If you are reasonably fit, active, and slim and yet still suffer from back pain, it may be that your spinal problems result from poor use of your back. Do you slouch from a saggy bed to a poorly designed, overstuffed sofa? Do you sit with your legs crossed? Do you always carry heavy bags on one side of your body? Is your toddler transported around slung across your hip? What about picking things up from the floor? It's easy to forget about safe lifting: *always* bend at the knees.

There are some simple and basic rules for using your spine with respect. Have a good, close look at what you sit on. Try to avoid deep sofas (the sort that look wonderful and feel terrible), or any chair that forces your spine to curve the wrong way. If you have no choice but to use these seats, always support your lower back with a small cushion or lumbar roll. Experts say that the greatest pressure to your spinal discs is caused by sitting in soft chairs for long periods of time. If you use a footrest, bend your knees rather than sitting with your legs stretched out straight in front of you.

When was the last time you saw a cat with a back problem? Probably never. Cats instinctively know the health benefits of stretching. Take some tips from the feline experts. If you are forced to sit for long periods of time (an hour or more), such as at your desk or behind the steering wheel, try taking frequent "stretch breaks." If you have some privacy, try the cat stretch. Get down on your hands and knees, with your hands pointing forwards. With elbows stiff, bend your knees and lower yourself down and back on your legs. Breathe deeply and relax into your stretch. It feels wonderful, and is great for shoulder and upper back tension.

"Don't use your back like a crane," as a New Zealand back-care campaign advised a few years ago. Take those words to heart. Whenever you pick something up, even if it's only a piece of lint off the carpet, *always bend your knees*. Don't ever bend forward from the waist with your knees locked and your legs straight. If you are carrying a heavy weight, carry it in front of you, tucked in close to your body.

Sometimes even sleeping can be a health hazard. You will spend a third of your life in bed, and what you sleep on can greatly affect how you feel for the other two thirds of your life. The ideal mattress supports your spine in the same position as if you were standing with good posture. Mattresses with mountain ranges and valleys are definitely no good. Generally, supportive mattresses need to be firm. However, many chronic back pain sufferers find relief by sleeping on a waterbed. What position you sleep in can also affect your spine. If you suffer from low back pain, the most beneficial positions for you to sleep in are either lying on your back with your knees raised, or curled up on your side in a semi-fetal position. Some people find it helpful to place a pillow between their knees when sleeping on their sides. Never lie flat on your back with your legs out straight, as this places great strain on your lower lumbar vertebrae.

"Keep fit" became a catch-phrase in the 1980s, and they're still words to live by. Exercise is beneficial for every aspect of the body, when done correctly. Incorrect exercising, on the other hand, can cause great damage to your body. Often it is the spine that bears the brunt of your unwise exercise.

American studies using magnetic resonance imaging (MRI) have shown that long-term jogging on hard surfaces causes microscopic fractures in the spinal bones and hip bone (femur). Remember, never be tempted to begin any type of exercise without at least 10 minutes of stretching and warm-up exercises.

Back-care experts recoil in horror at some of the exercise routines commonly performed in gyms around the country. Avoid head rolling exercises—rolling your head in clockwise and counter-clockwise circles. This can cause serious neck problems. If you want to perform toe-touching exercises from a standing position, go ahead. Just make sure that your knees are always bent slightly. Rigidly locked knees and straight legs endanger your lower back. Also, stand up *slowly* when you're through. Any exercise that involves twisting and bending simultaneously places you at risk of spinal injury. Finally, avoid doing straight leg sit-ups. Make sure that your legs are bent and raised at the knee, with your feet planted firmly on the floor.

Despite all your best intentions and prevention, there may be a time when you join the ranks of back pain statistics. If you require treatment, your first stop will usually be your doctor's office. Usually your doctor will then refer you for treatment to a physiotherapist, osteopath, or chiropractor. Traditionally, physiotherapy was the most likely treatment. These days, however, the unique spinal-care skills of osteopaths and chiropractors are fully recognized, and both osteopathy and chiropractic treatment are covered by Workers' Compensation and a number of insurance plans.

Chapter 4

Mind Matters

So far these pages have focused on two of the three most important prerequisites for staying well—sound nutrition and regular, appropriate exercise. Now it's time to focus on the third side of the triangle—mental and emotional harmony. Diet, exercise, and good mental health are interdependent. A perfect diet will not lead to optimum health if you lead the life of a sloth and suffer continual stress. Similarly, you could meditate from dawn until dusk, but if you exist on a junk food diet and never exercise, your body will eventually break down. Running several miles a day will not forestall a heart attack if your life is a relentlessly grueling series of stresses, which you cope with by binging on junk foods. So you see, no one side of the staying-well triad is of much use without the other two.

Stress

This has to be the catch-word of modern Western existence. Pick up any newspaper or magazine, turn on the television, or simply listen to the conversation between a few mothers or a group of business people, and you are bound to hear this word within the first few minutes. Chances are you're well aware of some form of stress within your own life, and of its detrimental effects. Still, doing something about it is another story.

What Exactly Is Stress?

Stress is caused by any change to which you must adjust. The most obvious stressful events you may encounter include changing jobs, moving, falling in or out of love, marrying or divorcing, becoming a parent, suffering the death of a loved one. Feelings of stress are triggered by three sources:

- The environment around you
- Your body
- Your mind (thoughts).

Environmental stress may be something as simple as extremes of weather, or it may result from problems with the environment in which you live—such as overcrowding and poor housing. Excessive work and time demands also fall into this environmental category of stress.

Bodily sources of stress include major physiological changes such as periods of rapid growth, adolescence, menopause, pregnancy, illness, poor nutrition, and lack of exercise.

The third major stress source is your mind—how you interpret and decide to cope with the changes occurring around you. This is the area of stress you can probably do the most to modify. The good news is that a few changes here will increase your ability to deal with the stressors in the other two categories, which may well be ongoing and unavoidable.

How Does Stress Affect Your Body?

Whenever your body interprets a situation as being stressful, it triggers an intricate chain of physiological reactions to allow it to deal with the stress. In many ways the body is still steeped in its primitive past, and when it comes to stress, your body responds in the same way as your cave-dwelling ancestors. For the cave dwellers, stress was usually a physical danger of some sort, such as being pursued by a hungry animal. Today, the human body still interprets stress as danger, and triggers the same physiological changes that allow you to stay and "fight" the danger, or to take "flight."

This reaction is known as the "fight or flight" response. At such moments bodily changes include an immediate and dramatic increase in adrenalin production (the hormone secreted by your adrenal glands, to sharpen all your senses). In turn, this increased adrenal function causes some major physiological processes to slow down. These include your digestion, growth, any tissue repair and healing occurring in your body, and your immune response. Simultaneously your heart begins to beat faster and your blood pressure increases—both responses to allow more oxygen to be delivered to your muscles, should they be required to move quickly in flight. Blood flow is redirected away from your extremities to your important muscles and organs. Your pupils dilate to improve your vision, and your hearing becomes more acute.

These physiological changes are designed to be of help to you. In a danger situation they may well allow you to take evasive action and stay alive. By staying and fighting or turning on your heels and running, you are taking some kind of decisive action that will end the immediate stress. When this happens, your body quickly gets the "all clear" message and returns to its normal pre-stress condition.

Now this is where the problem occurs for many twentieth century folks. If you find yourself living in the face of constant, seemingly unsolvable stress, your body never receives its all clear message. Instead it lingers on for days, weeks, or years in the "red alert" condition. When this happens, all those physiological changes that were designed to help you, end up harming you. Many of the chronic health problems prevalent in the West are the result of these stress-induced body changes. These include heart disease, high blood pressure, cancer, asthma, digestive problems, ulcers, constipation or irritable bowel syndrome, and mental or emotional disorders such as depression.

Some Common Symptoms of Excessive Stress

If you suffer from any of the following symptoms regularly, your body is probably trying to sound a stress alert:

- Anxiety
- Hostility and anger
- Irritability and resentment
- Irrational fears or phobias
- Obsessive, repetitive thoughts
- Muscle tension, particularly in the shoulders, neck, chest, and jaw
- Headaches, backaches, neckaches
- High blood pressure, chest pain, or palpitations
- Indigestion, excessive gas, abnormally large or small appetite
- Chronic constipation or diarrhea
- Tics or tremors
- Difficulty getting to sleep, restless sleeping, and early waking
- Physical weakness and exhaustion
- Low or no interest in sex
- Menstrual irregularities or complete lack of menstruation
- Feeling you need frequent cups of coffee, cigarettes, or alcohol to get through the day.

However, not all stress is bad for you. Some stress can be good for you, and in fact can help you to face challenges in your life more successfully. Feeling stressed just before taking an important exam is natural, and often the heightened awareness that results from the extra adrenalin pumping in your veins will help you meet your challenge more effectively. Stress only becomes a problem when it is ongoing and excessive, to the point of causing physical and emotional symptoms of imbalance (such as those listed above).

Each person has unique stress tolerance levels. If you have reached yours, it's time to take some serious evasive action, and learn how to minimize your stress or how to change your responses to that stress.

Some Simple Starting Points for Dealing With Stress

So you have finally decided enough is enough, and you're sick of the anxiety, sleepless nights, and joylessness of your life, but you're not quite sure just where to begin and what practical steps you can take to reduce your stress levels. The following are useful starting points.

Step One

Take a long, hard look at your life and your commitments. Is your life lived at breakneck speed, rushing from one commitment to another, never having time for yourself, for contemplation and relaxation? If your answer is yes, then your first plan of action has to be some serious commitment pruning. This often involves learning how to say no, which in turn involves a degree of assertiveness that many people lack. Women in particular have great difficulty coming to terms with the notion that they can turn down other people's requests for help. Traditionally, women are raised to fill the stereotypical roles of caregivers and nurturers—roles often filled at the expense of their own needs for time and space.

If you are a mother at home with children, maybe you could allocate yourself more time by alternating babysitting sessions with another mother. Maybe you need to make more demands on your partner for practical assistance around the home, and daycare sessions to allow yourself time out to pursue a hobby, go for a walk, or simply lock yourself away for a good sleep.

Mothers who also work outside the home face stresses of a different kind. Full-time mothers may have to cope with such problems as boredom, isolation, and lack of adult stimulation; working mothers face problems that often include the pressures of performing several different and demanding roles simultaneously, lack of adequate support structures, feelings of guilt at leaving pre-school children, and possibly the frustration of having to work for financial reasons, even when they would prefer to stay at home.

Step one, then, is a search for opportunities to open up space for yourself. Don't think of this as selfish. Think of it as tune-up time to keep yourself in top running condition for yourself and all the others who depend on you.

Step Two

When you are working (be it in a paid job, or unpaid mothering), do you allocate yourself adequate employment standards? You should try not to work longer than nine hours a day (obviously this is not possible if you have children), and set time aside for lunch breaks and tea breaks. You need at least a half-hour break in the middle of the day to allow for recharging of your batteries. Remember, too, that it's not healthy to have all work and no play—you need at least one and a half days off each week.

Step Three

Remember to eat! That might sound like strange advice, but it is surprising how many people get so caught up in the rush of everyday routine that they neglect to feed themselves regularly. Going for long periods of time without food, or starting the day without a decent breakfast, puts stress on your body. Irregular eating leads to wild fluctuations of blood sugar, which are usually accompanied by feelings of fatigue, weakness, irritability, headaches, sweating or shakiness, and depression.

Aim to start each day with a complex carbohydrate and protein breakfast (such as whole grain toast with fish or eggs), and then eat at least every three hours throughout the day. Snack on fresh fruit, nuts and seeds, whole grain bread with spreads such as peanut butter, guacamole, low- or non-fat yogurt, all-fruit jams, or cold meat. As some of these offer fat along with their nutrients, hold yourself to small (but satisfying) servings of peanut butter, avocado-based spreads, and meats. Try to avoid the temptation of quick pick-me-ups such as chocolate bars or cookies and cake. These concentrated sugar sources only exacerbate the problem of blood sugar fluctuations (as does reaching for a cup of caffeine).

Step Four

Along with remembering to eat comes remembering to sleep! Most people need around seven or eight hours' quality sleep a night. While it is possible to get into the habit of a late bedtime and still function during the day, your body is not getting the recuperation time it really needs. If you are having trouble sleeping, try some of the tips outlined on the subject of insomnia in Chapter 12.

Step Five

Regular aerobic exercise, as little as 20 minutes three times a week, will make a difference to your mental as well as physical health. Aerobic exercise stimulates the production of brain chemicals (endorphins), which help to elevate your mood and counteract feelings of stress and tension. Exercise will also help regulate your diet and contribute to a sound night's sleep.

Step Six

Practice some type of regular relaxation exercise, such as those outlined below. Consider breathing exercises, meditation, progressive relaxation, yoga, tai chi, or simply some relaxing activity such as a beach walk, a bath by candlelight, or a massage. A concentrated relaxation break will pay you back many times in increased productivity and well-being during your "on" times.

Step Seven

Remember that complementary therapies have a lot to offer in helping you deal with stress overload. In particular acupuncture, massage, and herbal medicine are noted for their effectiveness in this area. Ongoing emotional or physical stress greatly increases your body's requirements for a range of vitamins and minerals. In particular, your need for vitamins C and the B complex, and the minerals calcium and magnesium, increase dramatically. The following is a useful guideline for using nutritional supplements to help combat the ill effects of ongoing stress.

- Invest in a balanced time-release B complex formula, providing at least 50 mg of the major B vitamins. This can be taken two to three times daily with meals, depending on your current levels of stress.

- Your adrenal glands (your first-line responders to stress) require additional B5 (pantothenic acid) in order to maintain their hyper function. Add up to 1000 mg a day of B5, to be taken in conjunction with your balanced B complex.

- Vitamin C can be taken three times a day, in doses anywhere from 500 mg to several thousand milligrams. You know you have overdone the vitamin C if your stools become loose and urgent, in which case your dosage should be reduced slightly.

- Look for a multi-mineral formula containing magnesium, calcium, and zinc. Chelated or orotate minerals have the highest degree of absorbability. Aim for between 1000 to 1500 mg of calcium per day, with half this amount of magnesium. Minerals are best absorbed when taken on an empty stomach.

If you are pregnant, have a current medical condition, or are using medication, see your health care professional before self-prescribing a nutritional program.

Progressive Relaxation

Your mind and body function as one inextricably linked unit. Whatever happens in your mind is felt and reflected by your body. Conversely, bodily experiences affect your mind. It follows then that if you go through your days feeling stressed, anxious, and tense, your body is going to mirror these feelings in its structure, by becoming rigid, tense, and stiff. These bodily feelings of tension in turn increase your mental feelings of tension and anxiety.

Learning how to relax your body gives you a tool with which to relax your mind. A stress-free body means a stress-free mind. The following technique, known as progressive relaxation, has produced excellent results in the treatment of stress-induced disorders such as muscular tension, insomnia, irritable bowel syndrome, neck and back pain, high blood pressure, anxiety, and depression.

To practice this exercise, set aside one or preferably two 15-minute sessions per day. Take the phone off the hook, close the doors, and eliminate any possible interruptions! Lie comfortably on your bed or on the floor (or just sit in a comfortable high-backed chair with your head supported, if you're at work). You will work through the various muscle groups in your body, first tensing and then relaxing them, becoming aware of how different a relaxed muscle feels from a tense one.

Starting with your hands, curl your fists up into tight balls. Hold the tension for about seven seconds, before completely relaxing your hands for twenty to thirty seconds. Next repeat the same procedure, this time tensing the muscles in your forearms. Work on up the arms before repeating the process with your face, throat, and shoulders. Remember to tense the muscles as much as possible, and to notice the contrast when the muscles are relaxed. Next work with the muscles in your chest, stomach, and lower back, before finishing with the thighs, buttocks, calves, and lastly your feet. You can repeat the tensing-holding pattern for each muscle group twice, if you have the time. This will help you achieve and notice an even deeper state of relaxation.

Be patient—this is a skill to be learned and perfected like any other. When you first begin this exercise you will probably only be able to achieve partial relaxation. Persevere, and in time your efforts will be rewarded with a new-found sense of physical and emotional relaxation.

Do You Know How To Breathe?

That may seem like a silly question for someone who has spent an entire life performing this action! While it's true that all people breathe efficiently enough to stay alive, not so many of us breathe correctly for optimal health and well-being. Shallow breathing deprives your blood of valuable oxygen, which in turn means that your muscles and tissues are poorly oxygenated. This lack of oxygen can itself contribute to feelings of anxiety, depression, and fatigue.

Even something as fundamental as taking a breath is affected by stress and muscular tension. The next time you are feeling particularly tense, take a moment to pay attention to your breathing. You will probably notice that you are taking little, shallow, short breaths, breathing only from the upper part of your chest. This leaves two-thirds of your lung capacity sitting vacant and unused. The aim of this exercise is to teach you how to breathe deeply and efficiently, thus increasing your oxygen intake and counteracting feelings of anxiety.

Lie on your back on the floor with your knees bent slightly and your feet placed flat on the floor about one foot apart. Take a few moments to release any muscle tension that you are aware of (perhaps using a quick version of the progressive relaxation technique).

Place one hand on your abdomen, just above your navel, and your other hand on your chest. Slowly take a deep breath in through your nose, drawing the air down into your abdomen, causing your abdominal hand to rise up. Your chest will move only slightly, as your abdomen inflates. This is what a true breath feels like! Hold for a moment, then exhale completely in a smooth stream. After a few minutes of breathing this way, start to breathe in through your nose and out through your mouth. Focus all your attention on the feel and sound of breathing this way.

At first five to ten minutes of this deep breathing will probably be enough to make you feel slightly light-headed and hyperventilated. After a few weeks, though, you'll find you are able to perform this exercise for twenty minutes or more.

When you feel totally comfortable with this exercise, it's time to make this new way of breathing part of your daily existence, rather than just an exercise. Begin by breathing this way whenever you think of it during the day, most especially when you feel yourself tensing up. Gradually you will be able to adopt deep breathing on a permanent basis.

If you seriously want to learn new skills for "de-stressing," there are other effective techniques that are most probably being taught somewhere in your local community. These include meditation, yoga, tai chi, self-hypnosis, and creative visualization. Check your local library (which may have a community bulletin board) and high school (for a list of suitable night classes).

Chapter 5

Women and
Cigarette Addiction

There can't be one American woman alive who doesn't know that smoking is bad for you, that it can and does take lives. Yet thousands of women and men still take up this dirty, expensive, and self-destructive habit each year. Most women know of the link between smoking and lung cancer, heart disease, and circulatory disease. Not so many women know that smoking increases your chances of developing breast and cervical cancer, reduces your fertility, increases your chances of miscarrying or giving birth to a premature and underweight baby, causes premature menopause, and contributes to dramatic early aging in terms of skin wrinkling.

If you are using the contraceptive pill and smoking too, you increase your chances of developing circulatory disorders, which could kill you. Ninety-two percent of pill users who suffer a heart attack are smokers!

Smoking also increases your likelihood of developing osteoporosis. This condition, which mostly affects post-menopausal women, can see you fracturing bones from something as simple as coughing, or breaking an ankle bone from simply stepping from your car.

So you know the reasons for quitting, and you want to quit, but you don't know how to go about it. Don't give up before you even start. You can kick the habit like thousands of women before you. A few simple procedures can make your transition from your coughing days a less painful one.

How Do You Start To Kick the Habit?

A bit of aversion therapy may help. Take a good look at the hard facts regarding the effects of smoking on your precious body. Forget the trendy advertisements promising you social acceptance, blue skies, and glittering Caribbean oceans if you continue to smoke. The picture they portray couldn't be further from the truth. There is hardly a single part of your body that remains unaffected each time you light up.

Cigarettes cause damage to your lungs, heart, and cardiovascular system, your digestive system, your immune system, and your reproductive system. Watching our fat intake and worrying about cholesterol levels seem to be the health obsessions of the 1990s. If you're a smoker, you'll be fighting a losing battle. Cigarettes increase the cholesterol levels in your blood, at the same time decreasing the protective high-density fats, making heart attacks more likely. Smoking is responsible for 20 to 30 percent of heart disease, with smokers being three times more likely than non-smokers to have a heart attack. Cigarettes harden the walls of your arteries, making them less flexible and more prone to blockages. As well as stiffening, the artery walls are actually thickened by a layer of collagen. Narrow arteries are less efficient movers of blood. The heart muscle may become starved of oxygen and then cramp, causing painful angina. This same damage to the arteries reduces the flow of blood to the brain, greatly increasing your chances of suffering a stroke.

If you're a smoker reading this now and feeling sick with worry, don't despair. The good news is that it is never too late to do yourself a lifesaving favor. Stop smoking now, and in a year's time you will be 50 percent less likely to die of a heart attack. Ten years from now you will be at no greater risk than someone who has *never* smoked.

As if that isn't enough to worry about, your poor lungs also take a major battering from your addiction. Every time you have a cigarette, your lungs are exposed to a barrage of irritating chemicals that trigger inflammation and eventually scarring of the delicate tissues lining your airways and lungs. The least traumatic result of this is a marked propensity to catching colds and flus, bronchitis, and chronic sinusitis. However, after 20 or 30 years of smoking you have the very real likelihood of developing emphysema and also lung cancer (with an incidence that is nearly 14 times higher for women who smoke than for women who have never smoked).

If you treasure your teeth, you have another good reason to snub this habit. Smokers have a much higher incidence of periodontal disease. Gums bleed and recede, and teeth become loose and then fall out. While you do still have your teeth, they are stained and unattractive.

Smoking doubles your chances of developing a stomach ulcer—something to take seriously, especially if you're in a high-stress job, as prolonged stress itself predisposes you to stomach ulcers.

If you still manage to delude yourself that you are somehow immune to all the horrific smoking-induced diseases, take a look in the mirror and you will be confronted by another unpleasant accompaniment to smoking. Cigarettes age you. With the reduced supply of oxygen to your skin and the overall drying effect of cigarettes, your skin dries, withers, and wrinkles much more rapidly. If you smoke, your face at 40 will resemble the face of a 50- or even 60-year-old non-smoker. And you can forget all the promises of expensive rejuvenation creams—this damage occurs from the inside out.

Along with AIDS, cancer would have to be one of today's most feared killers. Reaching for your pack greatly increases the probability of your developing cancer of the lungs, mouth, bladder, and pancreas. Over 40 percent of bladder cancers are a direct result of smoking. Every cigarette that you put to your lips reduces your life expectancy by five and a half minutes.

It all makes pretty depressing reading so far, doesn't it? But knowing the facts may help you to overcome your addiction.

What of Your Children?

Many women smokers find that one of the greatest incentives to give up smoking is a genuine concern for the health of their children—the innocent passive smokers. The non-smoker who is forced to inhale cigarette fumes for long periods of time suffers the same detrimental effects as the smoker. A passive smoker in a smoky room for eight hours has a level of carbon monoxide in his or her body equivalent to having smoked five cigarettes—a particularly sobering thought if that passive smoker is your new baby or toddler.

Children of smoking parents also suffer from far more respiratory infections than children of non-smokers. They are admitted to the hospital for pneumonia and bronchitis more frequently; asthma and middle-ear infections are more common. Children of smokers are also shorter than average. Babies born to smoking parents are much more likely to die from crib death than "non-smoking" babies. Isn't all that enough to help you rush past the cigarette stand at the supermarket?

Why Do You Smoke?

You smoke because nicotine is one of the most addictive drugs in existence. Puffing on nicotine causes a feeling of being "up," partly due to its effect on your blood pressure (which increases when you have a cigarette) and heart rate, and partly due to a variety of hormones and body chemicals produced in response to the nicotine. Nicotine actually mimics some of the chemicals found in your brain, which are responsible for elevating your mood. Your liver is also affected by the drug, prompting it to elevate your blood sugar temporarily and cause you to feel energized.

Despite what the advertising moguls tell you, smoking low-tar cigarettes is not really a safe smoking option. The only safe option is stopping altogether. What tends to happen with low-tar-and-nicotine cigarettes is that you simply "drag" harder and smoke more cigarettes to give your body the same nicotine fix it is used to. These cigarettes also contain more of the other deadly chemicals found in cigarettes, including carbon monoxide, cyanide, and nitrogen gases. These chemicals actually increase your risk of developing heart disease and lung damage due to the increased oxygen deficit they induce.

So How Do You Stop?

If you really do want to stop smoking, you may be wondering just what the best way is to go about it. There is no best way. Some people find that cold turkey withdrawal is the only way for them. Others find that a gradual reduction over a period of weeks works.

Whichever method you choose, be aware that nicotine is a powerful drug, and it is almost certain that you will experience some kind of withdrawal symptoms along the way. These may include irritability, insomnia, tremors, headaches, poor concentration, and of course a craving for cigarettes! You will experience cravings for as long as it takes your body to detoxify and rid itself of the residues of nicotine stored in your fat cells and your liver. You can decrease your detoxification time by making sure that your fluid intake is high (not coffee or alcohol though), exercising frequently, and using additional methods of detoxification such as regular saunas.

Stopping (and staying stopped) may be less traumatic if approached in an ordered and systematic way. It often helps to practice for the big day, by gradually reducing your cigarettes day by day. Get a little notebook and record every cigarette you smoke. If you smoke 25 today, tomorrow smoke 24 and no more. Reduce by one a day, gradually getting down to one or two cigarettes a day. From here, the transformation to "non-smoker" is a relatively painless one. Try to hold out longer each day before reaching for your first light. There is evidence that shows that the earlier you light up, the more often you'll smoke during that day.

When the big day arrives and you declare yourself a non-smoker, take some practical action to show yourself your commitment is sincere. Try going through your house and clearing out every cigarette you find. Wash out your ashtrays and give them away (ideally to a non-smoking friend who can use them as coasters or art!). It may also be helpful to arrange your life to help you stay away from cigarettes. Take up a sport, sit in non-smoking areas in restaurants and other public places, open a special account and deposit every dollar you save by not smoking.

Try a little mind exercise—tell yourself not to think of a red rose. You'll find it almost impossible to keep the forbidden picture from your mind. The same applies during those first few difficult weeks, when you tell yourself desperately not to think of cigarettes. The most effective way to keep a thought from your mind is to focus actively on something else. When the craving for cigarettes starts, create diversions such as going for a walk, phoning a friend, or cleaning the car. Do anything except sit down to try not to think about cigarettes!

Diet and Nutrition

While you are reducing your intake of nicotine, pay particular attention to the quality (and quantity) of your diet. Cigarettes artificially elevate your blood sugar, and when you stop smoking there may be many times a day when low blood sugar makes you feel worse than you need to. To help avoid this, begin each day with a high-quality breakfast of complex carbohydrates and protein. For example, why not try cereal and fresh fruit; unsweetened granola, fruit, and yogurt; whole grain toast and eggs, fish, or cold meat; or buckwheat pancakes and mashed banana. The complex carbohydrates and protein are digested slowly, supplying a slow and sustained release of sugar to help you get through your morning without turning into a wicked witch.

Eat Little and Often

During the day have small, frequent snacks of good quality food. Avoid the trap of replacing the missing cigarettes with endless packets of peppermints or chocolate donuts. The sudden sharp burst of sugar they supply will help you feel better temporarily, but worse in the long run. All the extra calories won't do anything for your figure, except expand it alarmingly. Snack on fruit, nuts and seeds, whole grain bread and cheese or avocado, yogurt, cold meats, or rice crackers with peanut butter or unsweetened jam. If you feel really bad, chewing on a piece of natural licorice wood (available from some health food shops) will stabilize your blood sugar and support your adrenal glands (which will most probably be exhausted from the effects of smoking).

Smokers tend to have a mildly acidic body pH, and it is useful to consume a predominantly alkaline diet while you are cutting down (or out) your cigarettes. This has been scientifically proven to decrease your nicotine cravings. An alkaline diet involves high consumption of alkaline foods while at the same time cutting down on acid foods. Alkaline foods include most fruits and vegetables (especially green vegetables, lima beans, celery, and carrots), almonds, and millet. Note that fruits, when metabolized, produce an alkalinizing effect on the body, even though they may taste and look acidic. Acid foods form the basis of much of the modern Western diet, and include such foods as meat, wheat, sugar, and dairy products. The alkaline foods also tend to be high-fiber, low-fat foods which further aid in your body's process of detoxification.

There is a strong correlation between smoking and drinking coffee. Many smokers reach for a cigarette each time they have a cup of coffee. If you drink more than an occasional cup of coffee, it is important to cut down (and even cut out) your coffee drinking before you start to give up smoking. Try replacing your coffee with one of the many available herbal teas.

Nutritional Supplements for Giving Up Smoking

Heavy smokers invariably suffer from a range of nutritional deficiencies, particularly a lack of vitamins C, B, and A. Cigarettes block the absorption of these nutrients, or actively destroy them in the body—for example, each cigarette you smoke destroys 25 mg of your precious vitamin C. It is particularly helpful to use nutritional supplements as you go through withdrawal.

Vitamin C

Taken in the form of calcium ascorbate during your detoxification program, vitamin C will help to reduce your body's acidity and alkalinize your urine. While this does slow the excretion of nicotine through your urine, it also reduces cravings, and is particularly useful if you are suffering from overwhelming nicotine cravings as a result of detoxifying too rapidly. You need to take large amounts (about 1000 mg every two hours) for this to work.

The B Complex Vitamins

These will help you feel calmer and allay some of the irritability and insomnia you may experience, and you can be virtually certain that these "nervous system" nutrients are lacking in your body if you are a smoker. Use a high potency balanced B complex which supplies at least 50 mg of the major B vitamins, taken twice daily with food.

Calcium and Magnesium

Use a multi-mineral formula supplying substantial amounts of calcium and magnesium, balanced in the correct 2 to 1 ratio. Taken twice daily with food, these mineral relaxants will lessen withdrawal symptoms and prevent insomnia, so common with cigarette withdrawal.

Vitamin A

This is best taken in the beta-carotene form. Take up to 75,000 iu a day for the first few weeks after giving up smoking, then cut back to 25,000 iu a day. Vitamin A is an anti-oxidant and a powerful detoxifier, and helps the healing of the mucous membranes lining the throat, nose, and lungs.

Herbal Remedies

There are various herbal "calmers" available to ease your withdrawal pains. Simple herbal teas such as chamomile, valerian, and lemon balm can be drunk as and when you need their calming effects. Herbal nervous system strengtheners (nervines) are useful to take for the first couple of weeks after you stop smoking. These formulations usually contain combinations of such herbs as scullcap, valerian, hops, catnip, passion-flower, and chamomile.

Herbs are also useful as cleansers and detoxifiers, speeding and enhancing your body's ability to excrete residues of nicotine and other toxic chemicals stored in your body. Detoxifying teas can be made using dandelion root (dandelion coffee), red clover, or pau d'arco (all available in dried form from most health shops).

Homeopathic Remedies

There are several homeopathic remedies useful to lessen your craving. These include Avena, Caladium, Tabacum, and Nux Vomica. Tabacum is best used in the 3 c potency, with the other remedies most appropriate in the 30 c potency. Tabacum 3 c is useful to take whenever your craving for tobacco threatens to thwart your good intentions—simply suck a couple of the tablets and wait for your craving to leave you.

Acupuncture

Many women find that their ability to stop smoking has been greatly enhanced by a few sessions of acupuncture, before and during their withdrawal. Treatment usually involves the insertion of a small stud needle into the "stop smoking" point in the ear. This is then covered with tape, and stays in place for about a week. You can stimulate the needle yourself whenever you have a craving. General acupuncture treatment is also given, in particular to strengthen the lungs and calm the patient.

Whatever methods you choose to use to overcome your addiction, the ultimate tool is your own strength of mind and determination. Be proud of yourself and your commitment to a healthier future. Within a few months your new-found vitality and sense of well-being will be confirmation enough that the struggle has been worth the trouble!

Chapter 6

Contraception—
To Have Not

Compared with your grandmother, you have it made when it comes to choosing when to have or not to have babies. However, scientists still haven't invented the perfect contraceptive. No contraceptive (short of celibacy) can promise 100 percent protection, and you trade off the inconvenience of barrier methods for the potential health risks of hormonal contraceptives. Work continues on developing the male contraceptive pill, but its release still appears to be years away.

So what contraceptive choices do you have? The options can be categorized into four groups:

- Barrier methods, such as condoms, the diaphragm, and the cervical cap. Although not strictly a barrier contraceptive, Intre-Uterine Devices (IUDs) can also be placed in this category.
- Local chemicals, such as spermicidal foams and gels.
- Hormonal preparations, such as the oral contraceptive pill, the progestin-only "mini-pill," and Depo-Provera.
- Natural family planning methods, which involve charting fertility and abstaining or using other contraceptives during the fertile days.

Barrier Methods

Condoms

Until recently, condoms were considered to be the poorer cousins of contraception. They were the butt of locker-room jokes, and were considered to be the sole domain of the fumbling adolescent. However, with the media now urging a return to condoms as protection against AIDS and other sexually transmitted diseases (STDs), sales have rocketed. A growing awareness of the drawbacks and dangers of the contraceptive pill and IUDs has also boosted a return to the humble condom.

If used consistently and in accordance with instructions, condoms offer extremely reliable contraception, without any side-effects. They also offer the most reliable protection against AIDs and STDs (short of not having sex at all).

So How Do You Use a Condom Effectively?

Condoms work if you use them *every* time you have intercourse, and if you put them on *prior* to any kind of genital-to-genital contact. A man often has sperm on the tip of his penis long before orgasm occurs, and theoretically this semen can impregnate you even if it only comes into contact with the outer area of your vagina.

Make sure that the condoms you use have not passed their expiration date, and that they are a recognized brand that meets health department standards. Any condoms you buy from a pharmacist will be approved. Even if you buy the best kind of condoms, there are a few circumstances that may make them less than reliable. Store your condoms in a cool place, as heat can warp the latex, making it more likely to tear. If you need additional lubrication during intercourse, don't use vaseline or any other petroleum-based lubricants, as these weaken the rubber. Instead, use a proper personal lubricant such as K-Y jelly.

After ejaculation, the penis should be withdrawn almost immediately to prevent the condom from slipping off as the penis softens and shrinks. Before withdrawing, grasp the condom firmly around the base. Once the condom has been removed, keep the penis well away from your vagina.

Condoms can be expensive, especially if you have an active sex life. However, they can often be obtained by prescription from your doctor, and this may work out as a cheaper option.

The Diaphragm

The diaphragm looks like a mini latex UFO with a rigid rim. It is filled with spermicide and then placed high in the vagina to fit around the cervix. It works in two ways: by providing a mechanical barrier to prevent semen from getting through to the cervix, and by holding the spermicide up against the cervix to kill off any particularly determined sperm that manage to bypass the obstacle. Diaphragms are effective contraceptives when they are properly fitted and used as instructed. They offer around 98 percent protection against pregnancy. If you want to use a diaphragm, it must be fitted by your gynecologist or family planning clinic doctor to ensure that the correct size is used. Once you are using your diaphragm, you must go back for a refitting if you lose or gain more than ten pounds of weight at any stage.

Besides protecting against pregnancy, diaphragms offer other advantages too. They are useful to hold back menstrual flow, and they make lovemaking more aesthetically pleasant during your period. There also seems to be some kind of protective effect against cervical and vaginal infections among women using diaphragms.

Not all women can have a diaphragm safely fitted, however. If you have a uterine prolapse or a tipped uterus (retroverted or anteflexed), you need to use another contraceptive method. Some women find the diaphragm messy and unpleasant to use, and this form of contraception is no good if you dislike touching your own genitals.

Cervical Cap

This wonderful device looks like an outsized rubber thimble. It is filled with spermicide and then fitted snugly right over your cervix, thus blocking the entry of any sperm. The cap is held tightly in place by suction, and must be left in for about eight hours following intercourse. However, many women leave their caps in place for several days, providing safe, ongoing, and convenient contraception.

As is the case with your diaphragm, you will need to have your cap personally fitted by your gynecologist or family planning clinic doctor. Some of the smaller clinics may be unable to provide this service, as the cap has never been enthusiastically promoted by manufacturers or doctors. Because it is inexpensive to produce, and lasts for a long time, it is a low-profit item for manufacturers who could instead be churning out millions of condoms or tubes of spermicide with a bulk turnover.

When it comes to effectiveness, the cap rates about as high as the diaphragm. It has no detrimental health effects, and can be inserted hours before intercourse (although spermicide must be reapplied if inserted more than three hours before intercourse).

Spermicides

Spermicides are available as creams, foams, or jelly. They are usually recommended to be used with some other form of contraception such as a condom, cap, or diaphragm. Spermicides are inserted high into the vagina to cover the cervix prior to sexual intercourse. They work in two ways: first they provide a physical barrier preventing sperm from entering the cervix; second they kill any sperm they come in contact with.

Spermicides have no side-effects (other than on the occasional woman who is allergic to them), and greatly boost the effectiveness of your barrier method of birth control. They offer the additional benefit of increased protection against sexually transmitted diseases such as gonorrhea and genital herpes. Spermicides also seem to decrease the incidence of less serious infections such as *trichomonas* and *monilia* (thrush).

IUD (Intra-Uterine Device)

If you are thinking of having an IUD fitted—don't. If you already use an IUD, think carefully about alternatives. This method of contraception has caused untold pain, suffering, and infertility in thousands of women around the world.

An IUD is a tiny, strangely shaped piece of plastic or copper with a tail string hanging off it that is inserted into your uterus, where it remains for as long as you wish to avoid pregnancy. It is still not understood exactly how IUDs work. One theory is that the IUD somehow prevents the fertilized egg from implanting in the uterus. Another is that the IUD dislodges the fertilized egg shortly after it has implanted, like a mini-abortion.

If you wear an IUD, your chances of developing pelvic inflammatory disease (PID), or a milder but still dangerous uterine infection, increase quite dramatically (some authorities claim by up to 900 percent). PID hospitalizes thousands of IUD users every year. PID can, and often does, lead to infertility, or to forced hysterectomy. If you have never had children, or you are young (under 20 years old), your risk of PID from an IUD is greatly increased.

Your troubles can start from the moment of insertion. Inserting the IUD can perforate your uterus (some studies show rates of up to eight perforations per 1000 insertions). You should never have an IUD fitted on your first visit to the doctor, as there are several preliminary checks you should have first. These include a physical examination, a blood test for anemia, a pap smear, and a test for gonorrhea. These tests must rule out pregnancy and diseases or abnormalities of your uterus which could cause serious complications if an IUD were fitted.

It's true that IUDs offer effective and convenient contraception, but at a very high price in terms of the potential risks to your health and long-term fertility. The number of women who die from IUD-induced complications is small. The number of women who experience problems serious enough to require hospitalization is quite high, however, ranging from around one in 100 to one in 300 per year.

What Kind of Problems Might You Encounter From an Iud?

Apart from PID, you may encounter a series of other difficulties. An IUD can increase your blood loss during your monthly period, sometimes tripling your flow. It can also increase the length of your period by up to four extra days. If you already have heavy periods, this could be potentially harmful for you, resulting in iron deficiency anemia. If you have painful periods now, the symptoms will be greatly compounded. IUD wearers have very painful periods, with lower abdominal and lower back cramps.

Like any other contraceptive, IUDs are not infallible. If you conceive while you still have an IUD in place, your chances of having a potentially life-threatening ectopic pregnancy are increased about tenfold—1 in 30

IUD wearers as opposed to 1 in 250 in non-IUD wearers. A pregnancy is ectopic when the fertilized egg implants itself somewhere outside of the uterus, usually in a fallopian tube. These pregnancies end with severe pain, loss of the baby, and often ruptured fallopian tubes and resulting infertility. Even if your pregnancy is not ectopic, you will have reason for concern if you are still wearing your IUD. About 50 percent of all "IUD pregnancies" will end in miscarriage, and the risk of septic abortions (infected miscarriages) is substantial.

Even if you do make it through your years of IUD use without any of these horrendous occurrences, there is much evidence to show that your future fertility may well be affected (even if you never suffered from PID). I, personally, would strongly advise women not to risk their fertility, and indeed their lives, for the sake of supposedly convenient contraception. Think seriously about a diaphragm, condoms, or a cap, and safeguard your health and well-being.

Hormonal Contraception

The contraceptive pill (combined estrogen/progesterone), the progestin-only "mini-pill," and the hormonal injection Depo-Provera, all fall in this category.

The Oral Contraceptive Pill (OCP)

The oral contraceptive pill (commonly called "the pill") consists of a combination of synthetic estrogen and progesterone. The pill imposes an artificial hormone balance that literally tricks your body into thinking it is already pregnant. The pill inhibits the release of two pituitary gland hormones that stimulate the ovaries to release an egg each month. No egg means no chance of pregnancy. Not content to stop there, the pill also changes your vaginal mucus, making it thick and impenetrable to sperm.

When the pill first hit the shelves in the fifties and sixties, it was hailed as a modern miracle and the perfect solution to fertility control. While there is no doubt that it offers one of the highest rates of protection against pregnancy, thirty-odd years of pill use have now shown that this "miracle" is not without its drawbacks and potentially serious side-effects.

What Are the Side-Effects?

The side-effects from taking the pill are numerous, ranging from annoying problems such as decrease in sex drive and weight gain through to life-threatening problems such as heart failure, stroke, and thrombosis. In general, the longer you take the pill, the more at risk you are of serious health problems. You are especially at risk if you are over 35, smoke, and are overweight.

When first starting to use the pill, it is quite common to experience some "minor" side-effects such as breast tenderness, an increase in normal vaginal discharge (and possibly thrush), weight gain, fluid retention, headaches, nausea, and vomiting. Using the pill can also increase your susceptibility to urinary tract infections and vaginal thrush, bronchitis, and viral infections such as chicken pox and colds. Gall bladder and liver disease is also more commonly seen among pill users, as are benign and cancerous tumors of the liver.

The whole question of cancer and the contraceptive pill is a complex and still largely unresolved one. Endometrial and ovarian cancer rates for pill users are actually lower than rates for other women. Does the pill contribute to the development of cancer of the cervix? The answer is still a confusing "we don't know." A 1985 World Health Organization study reported a 53 percent increase in cervical cancer among women who used the OCP for more than five years. At first sight the figure seems alarming, and it may indeed prove to be so, but the results are hard to interpret clearly because of the difficulty of keeping all the variables in the study under control—in particular, the sexual history of the participants.

Besides cancer, the other main area of concern with pill use is its potentially lethal effects on the circulatory system. Circulatory problems such as clotting abnormalities, heart attacks, and strokes have been the most responsible for pill-related deaths. Pill users between the ages of 15 and 34 are four times more likely to die from circulatory disorders than other women. Between the ages of 34 and 44 the risk escalates dramatically to a rate of ten times greater than the rate for women who do not use the pill. If you have been taking the pill for five years and smoke 25 or more cigarettes a day, your risk of dying from a heart attack is a whopping 20 to 40 times greater than the rate for women who neither smoke nor take the pill.

Thrombosis, or clots in the blood, is one of the most serious and real threats posed by the contraceptive pill. Your blood has the miraculous capability of clotting itself whenever you are cut, so that you don't bleed to death. These clotting factors are increased whenever you have high blood estrogen levels such as during pregnancy and of course when taking the pill. Women taking the pill have larger numbers of sticky platelets than normal—these are the cells that plug your wounds and prevent excessive bleeding.

Other more minor, but still disturbing, problems may arise with pill use. Pill-induced depression is very real and surprisingly common, especially among women using low-estrogen pills with high amounts of progesterone. These pills produce hormonal changes similar to those that you experience in the week or so before the onset of a period—the time when tension, irritability, depression, and anxiety are common. Whereas these emotional symptoms of PMS pass in a few days or a week, the pill-induced emotional changes are with you all month long.

While weight obsession and dieting disorders continue to become more and more prevalent among Western women, little thought is given to what role the contraceptive pill plays in this constant battle with weight gain. The pill does cause weight gain in a large proportion of users. This is partly because of the appetite-increasing effects of the synthetic progesterone it contains, and partly because of the fluid-retaining effects of the estrogen. In some women the estrogen also causes an increase in the "feminine" fat deposits; for example, on the hips, thighs, and breasts.

Don't Consider Using the Pill if . . .

- You are a cigarette smoker, especially if you are older than 35 years.

- You have a tendency to develop blood clots, or if you have a familial tendency to heart disease, high blood pressure, and high blood cholesterol.

- You have had cancer of the breast, uterus, cervix, or liver, or if you suffer from fibrocystic breast disease.

- You are pregnant or breastfeeding.

- You are under 18 or over 50 years old (or over 35 if you smoke).

- You suffer from bad headaches, migraines, diabetes, gall bladder problems, varicose veins, epilepsy, depression, chronic cystitis, asthma, or chronic vaginal infections.

The Pill and Nutritional Consequences

The pill also detrimentally affects your body's absorption, metabolism, utilization, and storage of a range of essential vitamins and minerals. Many pill users complain of a gradually worsening depression and loss of morale when taking the pill. This may well be the result of pill-induced changes in their absorption and utilization of the vitamin B_6—the synthetic estrogen blocks the absorption of this vitamin. B_6 deficiency retards the processing of some of the amino acids that affect your brain and are responsible for keeping you feeling happy and calm. If you are on the pill and feeling uncharacteristically depressed, supplementing your diet with a balanced B complex vitamin containing at least 50 mg of B_6 may help.

Remember, too, that you get vitamins from your food! Check Chapter 2 on nutrition and include plenty of vitamin B-rich foods in your daily diet.

Vitamin B_6 is not the only B vitamin to be depleted with continuous use of the pill: B_1 (thiamine), B_2 (riboflavin), B_{12} (cobalamin), and B_9 (folic acid) are all commonly deficient in pill users. In particular, B_9 deficiency can have serious consequences, with anemia and an increased susceptibility to cervical dysplasia as two of its more serious results. If you take the pill, I would strongly advise you to make a balanced B complex supplement a daily addition to your diet, to help safeguard against these common pill-induced deficiencies.

Vitamin C also takes a battering from the pill. Women who use this contraceptive are almost universally found to have low levels of vitamin C in their body. This is partly because of the high blood copper levels which the pill causes. The more copper you have circulating in your blood, the more vitamin C your body needs to function normally. The synthetic hormones also decrease your body's natural ability to absorb this vitamin from your food. Take a moment to read up on vitamin C again (in Chapter 2), and ponder the consequences of a deficiency of this vitamin.

There are also some plausible (but as yet scientifically unproven) theories that link vitamin C deficiency with increased risk of thrombosis (blood clots) and heart disease. It is best to take 1500 to 2000 mg of vitamin C daily, preferably in a supplement that also supplies bioflavinoids to enhance its absorption. Be generous with fresh fruits and vegetables to ensure a high dietary intake, too. As vitamin C supplements have the effect of increasing the uptake of estrogen in the gut (making your low-dose pill act more like a high-dose one), it is advisable to take vitamin C supplements at least four hours before or after taking the pill.

The fat-soluble vitamins (A, E, D, and K) are also affected if you take the pill because of its effect on your liver. Fat-soluble vitamins are processed and prepared for use in your liver, and the estrogen contained in the pill reduces its capacity to perform these functions. Vitamin E is universally acknowledged by nutritional experts as the vitamin *par excellence* when it comes to safeguarding against cardiovascular disease. It may well partly be the deficiency of this vitamin that contributes to the dramatically increased incidence of this type of disease in women who take the pill. Compensate for your body's inefficient processing of fat-soluble vitamins by supplementing with up to 800 iu of vitamin E daily, and including liberal amounts of E-rich foods in your diet (see the table on p. 60). Read the section on vitamin E in Chapter 2 before embarking on a supplementation regime.

When it comes to minerals, the most common finding in pill users is an abnormally high level of copper circulating in their blood, and a correspondingly low level of zinc. Copper and zinc have an inverse relationship—that is, when one is high the other is low. You need zinc to help you utilize those B vitamins which you will be taking. Zinc is essential for the digestion, the immune system, wound healing, skin, and a healthy reproductive system. You need about 50 mg of this supplement daily. Many of the good quality B complexes available here also contain elemental zinc to enhance the absorption and utilization of the B vitamins.

So, if you still want to use the pill, take steps to reduce the possibilities of side-effects. Eat a well-balanced diet, paying particular attention to an avoidance of saturated fats (to reduce your increased risk of cardiovascular disease) and refined carbohydrates (because of your decreased ability to process sugars properly). Definitely don't smoke. Exercise aerobically at least three times a week, for 20 to 30 minutes at a time. Invest some money and time in a daily nutritional supplement regime of vitamins B, C, E, and zinc. Have regular pap smears and blood pressure readings, and think of changing your contraception when you reach your late forties.

The "Mini-Pill"

The progestin-only "mini-pill" supplies synthetic progesterone, but no estrogen. Many women using this type of pill still ovulate each month, but by changing the consistency of the cervical mucus the pill still prevents pregnancy. The mini-pill causes the cervical mucus to become thickened and more acidic, thus rendering it particularly inhospitable to sperm. Should the sperm still manage to negotiate the "mucus trap" and make their way to your uterus, the mini-pill will still prevent pregnancy due to its effects on the lining of your uterus (endometrium). The endometrium is affected by the progestin, and is unable to support the implantation of a fertilized egg.

The mini-pill has a theoretical effectiveness rate of around 97 percent, compared to the combined pill effectiveness rate of around 99 percent. Of the side-effects experienced when using the mini-pill, the most commonly experienced for most women is menstrual irregularity. The risk of ovarian cysts is also greater for women who use the mini-pill, with some studies showing an increased incidence up to 200 percent. If you become pregnant while using the mini-pill, your pregnancy is more likely to be ectopic (occurring in a fallopian tube instead of in the uterus).

The mini-pill contains no estrogen and is therefore a preferred choice of hormonal contraception for women in whom estrogen use is contraindicated.

Depo-Provera

Depo-Provera is a synthetic progesterone, administered by injection, which provides protection against pregnancy for a three-month period. Depo prevents pregnancy by preventing ovulation, thickening the cervical mucus, and thinning the lining of the uterus, which makes it less hospitable for a fertilized egg. The injection is one of the most effective of all forms of contraception.

Depo-Provera has been surrounded by much controversy and is the subject of ongoing research regarding its potential, if any, for causing an increase in the risk of cancer, with some studies indicating that it may be associated with a greater risk of breast cancer in women under 25 years of age. Until long-term human studies have been carried out, the risk of cancer remains undeterminable.

One drawback of the injection is that once it has been administered, neither the positive effect of contraceptive protection nor the negative side-effects that some women experience can be "undone" until the injection wears off over a three-month period. Typical side-effects include altered menstruation, with irregular periods, heavy periods, or no periods at all commonly experienced. Weight gain (in 50 percent of women), headaches, abdominal bloating, and mood changes are other common side-effects. Finally, it can take up to a year for normal menstruation and fertility to return after you stop the injection—a factor that you should keep in mind if you plan to start a family after using this form of contraception.

Natural Family Planning

Natural family planning, sometimes called the rhythm method, used to be the domain of Catholics (forbidden to use contraceptives by their church), or hippies bent on doing everything the natural way. However, over the last few years there has been an increase in the number of other couples learning this method of fertility control. Natural family planning requires a commitment to learning about your fertility, and to observing and becoming more aware of the changes taking place in your body in the different stages of your cycle. It also requires a degree of self-control, because there are several days each month when intercourse is unsafe (unless of course you choose to use another contraceptive method such as a condom).

It is quite remarkable that your body can only conceive during a 12- to 36-hour period out of the whole month! When you release an egg (ovulation), it is only receptive to fertilization for these few hours. Taking into account the 3- to 5-day lifespan of an ejaculated sperm, and a variability in the exact time at which you ovulate, you actually come up with a "safe" time of around 18 days each month.

How do you determine when you ovulate? There are three signs to track:

- Detect changes in your vaginal mucus. When you ovulate, the mucus becomes slippery and copious, like raw egg white.

- Record your body temperature daily. Your temperature drops very slightly just before you ovulate, and then rises for about three days after you ovulate.

- Calculate your fertile periods by recording your menstrual cycle dates. This is probably the least reliable of the three methods.

Natural family planning has a higher failure rate than most of the other contraceptive methods. It also requires perseverance and self-discipline, and is only appropriate for couples in a committed, caring relationship.

Chapter 7

Planning for Your Pregnancy

Consciously planning the conception of your baby is a choice that women have been able to make only in relatively recent times. In previous generations women spent their lives struggling with pregnancy after pregnancy, with little realistic opportunity to create space and plan for each conception. Today's women have the advantages of being able to elect the timing of childbearing, and of having access to a huge amount of scientific and medical information regarding pregnancy.

The fetus is at its most vulnerable and is most easily damaged during the first eight to 10 weeks of pregnancy—a time when many women are not even aware they are pregnant. During the first three months of pregnancy your baby increases its mass by 2.5 million times, and this is accompanied by organization and differentiation of all its body cells. It is during these first critical months that abnormalities can occur.

It is not uncommon for women to continue taking their birth control pills (when, unknown to them, they have already failed!), to continue smoking, drinking, having X-rays, exposing themselves to potentially dangerous environmental chemicals, and taking medication, all during the critical first weeks of carrying a child.

Conscious conception involves making a decision to conceive a baby, often some months before actually setting out to do so. During the weeks and months leading up to conception you and your male partner actively undertake a commitment to becoming as fit, healthy, and nutritionally sound as is possible. This means:

- Weaning yourself and your partner off all potentially toxic drugs, including coffee and alcohol; social drugs such as marijuana, cocaine, and all other hard drugs; and prescription drugs including supposedly innocuous substances such as aspirin, panadol, and painkillers.
- Taking stock of all the potentially toxic chemicals you and your partner are exposed to, and then avoiding exposure as much as possible. This includes, for example, the use of chemical herbicides in the garden; exposure to lead if you are restoring an old

house that contains lead-based paints; exposure to lead from hobbies such as pottery or leadlights; or using pesticides around the house.

- Avoiding workplace contaminants and hazards. The most common and potentially dangerous include exposure to heavy metals such as lead, cadmium, mercury, copper, and arsenic (all of which have been implicated as causal factors in sterility and birth defects); acids such as those used in the manufacture of computer components; and radiation.

- Assessing the health of yourself and your partner. Treat any health problems that you are already aware of. Take care of any surgery or dental work you may need, before you try to conceive. Optimize your diet and nutrient intake and lose any excess weight.

- Checking that you (the woman) have immunity to rubella (confirmed through a blood test), and that your blood pressure is within a normal range. Ask for a hemaglobin and iron reading from the blood test to check that you are free from iron deficiency anemia.

- Examining your fitness levels. Do you tire easily and get out of breath simply climbing the two flights of stairs to your office? If so, you need to start improving your fitness now.

- Coming off the contraceptive pill and using an alternative form of contraception for at least three to six months before trying to conceive. The pill changes your body chemistry profoundly, affecting your nutritional status, immune function, and liver function. One of its most consequential effects, in terms of detrimental effect on your planned pregnancy, is its alteration of the copper and zinc levels in your blood (see Chapter 6 on contraception).

Stop Smoking

The research is absolutely irrefutable. Smoking can seriously damage every stage of reproduction, from the moment of conception, through the nine months of pregnancy, during the birth, and well into childhood. If you smoke, you will find it more difficult to become pregnant, and when you do conceive, your pregnancy will have a 25 percent higher risk of ending in miscarriage. Even after these risky early months, there is still a greatly increased possibility of premature birth.

So, if you are planning to conceive a baby, one of the most important and valuable things you can do for your child is to stop smoking *before* conception (see Chapter 5 on cigarette addiction for more information).

How Does Smoking Damage a Baby?

Your smoking will produce a lighter than normal baby. Low birth weight babies have a much higher risk of dying at or shortly after birth (40 times greater risk). Your baby will not only weigh less, but will also be physically smaller, that is, shorter, with a smaller head circumference, narrower shoulders, and a smaller chest. The effects of exposure to cigarettes while in the womb can slow your child's physical, mental, and emotional development right through until the age of 11.

All the 2000-plus toxic chemicals that you inhale when you smoke are passed through the placenta to your unborn child. Cadmium and cyanide affect your baby's utilisation of essential nutrients, leading to possible brain damage and abnormal cell growth. Carbon monoxide inhibits the delivery of oxygen and nutrients to your baby, compounding the effects of cadmium and cyanide.

If you smoke during pregnancy (and when your baby is an infant), your child has a 40 percent greater chance of dying within its first year of life. There is conclusive evidence that babies of smoking mothers are at greater risk of dying of crib death or sudden infant death syndrome (SIDS).

Even if you stop smoking during the nine months of pregnancy, your newborn is still at risk if you or your partner smokes after birth. Babies are detrimentally affected by passively inhaling the smoke in the air around them. Your baby will also receive nicotine through your breast milk if you smoke during the months of breastfeeding.

What About Alcohol?

There are volumes of studies illustrating the damaging effects of heavy alcohol consumption (more than five drinks a day) during pregnancy. These include increased incidence of stillbirth and premature birth, and an increased number of physical, intellectual, and emotional abnormalities. But when it comes to the question of complete abstinence versus moderate drinking, the authorities seem to differ. Some studies show risks to the unborn child with alcohol consumption as low as two drinks a week, while other studies indicate that this level of consumption causes no problems.

Every time you have an alcoholic drink your unborn baby gets the same drink via the placenta. While your mature liver quickly breaks down and detoxifies the alcohol, your baby's tiny liver is unable to perform this function as effectively. This means that your child keeps the alcohol in his or her system for up to 24 hours. Because research has been unable to establish a level of safe alcohol consumption during pregnancy, it is widely recommended that you abstain from alcohol completely while you are pregnant.

When you are planning your pregnancy, it is also a good idea to stop drinking (or drastically reduce your alcohol intake) for the weeks or months before conception. Studies have shown that women who drink daily before conception tend to have smaller babies. Your partner doesn't get off scot-free here either. There is evidence showing a strong connection between your male partner's alcohol consumption and the weight of your baby at birth. A recent study at the University of Washington looked at couples where the female abstained from alcohol and the male drank regularly. Where the men consumed as little as two drinks a day, the birth weight of the offspring was about six ounces lower than that of babies born to couples where the father drank only occasionally.

And Coffee?

Coffee is one of the most frequently consumed sources of caffeine, along with tea, chocolate, and Cola drinks. Coffee consumption only becomes a problem during pregnancy if you consume more than three or four cups a day. You can enjoy the occasional cup of drip coffee or a couple of cups of instant coffee each day without it affecting your baby.

Eating Right—Preparing Yourself Nutritionally

If you are well nourished when you conceive, your baby will be healthier. Your body will be stronger and better able to withstand the rigors of pregnancy, and it will have better reserves of nutrients with which to meet the demands of your growing child. A crop is only as good as the soil from which it springs, and the same holds for producing healthy babies. Studies going back as far as the 1940s show that malnutrition in the parents before conception (causing possible damage to the egg and sperm) is even more damaging to the fetus than that occurring after conception.

The healthy eating guidelines outlined in Chapter 2 provide a sound basis. Although these principles are useful for everyone, there are some nutrients that are particularly crucial for you before and during your pregnancy. These include calcium and magnesium, iron, folic acid, and zinc.

Calcium

Few women obtain the RDA of 1000 mg of calcium a day. Even fewer provide their bodies with the greatly increased calcium requirements of pregnancy. When you are pregnant, you are growing a whole new skeleton, created largely from calcium. If your diet fails to provide adequate daily calcium, your baby will simply drain the required calcium from your bones. If you have more than one pregnancy with this net calcium loss, you could well find yourself with osteoporosis later in life. During pregnancy you need to obtain 1500 mg of calcium each day from your food and mineral supplements.

Magnesium

Most dietary magnesium comes from whole grains and green leafy vegetables. Magnesium deficiency is common during pregnancy, when your daily requirement rockets to at least 450 mg. Preeclampsia (a potentially life-threatening disorder that produces high blood pressure and fluid retention during pregnancy) is more common in magnesium-deficient women. Your calcium supplement should be balanced with one part magnesium for every two parts of calcium. If it contains 400 mg of calcium, there should also be 200 mg of magnesium.

Iron

Iron deficiency anemia is extremely common among women in the reproductive years. If you are planning a pregnancy, it is a good idea to have your iron levels checked before you conceive. If they are low, you can then set about boosting your supplies with iron-rich foods and supplements. Approximately one-fifth of women who become pregnant have no or very limited stores of iron. When you are pregnant your iron requirement increases more than 100 percent to 30–60 mg a day. During pregnancy, not only do you have to furnish the iron requirements of your child, but at the same time your body manufactures a large amount of new blood as your blood volume increases.

Folic Acid

During pregnancy your requirements for this B complex vitamin double to about 800 mg a day. If your increased needs aren't met, you could encounter a range of problems, such as increased incidence of miscarriage, early birth, and birth defects (see pp. 40-41). Start increasing your folate stores well before conception by eating plenty of raw or lightly steamed green leafy vegetables, and fruit, and by using a balanced B complex supplement daily.

Zinc

If you are a vegetarian, your zinc supplies may well be low. This is because the most absorbable supply of zinc comes from red meat and seafood. The normal RDA for zinc increases to about 15 mg when you are pregnant. (See Chapter 2, p. 57, for further information on zinc and pregnancy.)

Using Fertility Awareness To Aid Conception

Learning to recognize your fertile time and the exact day of your ovulation is a useful way of optimizing your chances of conceiving if you are having trouble doing so. Having unprotected intercourse on the day before or on the exact day of ovulation will greatly increase your likelihood of conceiving. Some research indicates that by manipulating the timing of your conception you can load the dice in favor of conceiving a girl or a boy. This is because of the changes in your vaginal mucus at different times of your cycle and the effect the mucus has on any sperm swimming in your vagina. However, this research is not totally conclusive, and there are many other variables known to affect sex determination, including parental age, frequency of intercourse, and even your socio-economic group!

Around the time of your ovulation, your vaginal mucus is particularly hospitable for both sperm carrying an X chromosome (which will result in the conception of a girl) and those carrying a Y chromosome (resulting in a male child). However, because the Y sperm are lighter than the X sperm, they are able to move more rapidly to the waiting egg, thus increasing the chances of conceiving a male baby through a single act of unprotected intercourse on or just after ovulation.

If you want to conceive a girl, the advice is to have intercourse two or three days before you ovulate. At this time your vaginal mucus is more acidic and favors the survival of the more acid-resistant, X-carrying sperm. Remember, though, this is far from an exact science!

Chapter 8

Health Problems in Pregnancy

For many women, pregnancy is a time of supreme happiness and good health. Hormones cause a radiance of skin and hair and a general bloom of well-being for all to see. Increased blood volume and flow improve circulation, and the cold hands and feet you may have suffered for years are suddenly pink and warm again. Skin problems such as acne, eczema, and psoriasis may magically disappear for nine glorious months. This idyllic state of health is wonderful for those women whose bodies seem to have been designed with absolute perfection for the process of reproduction.

However, not all women are so lucky. You may have the misfortune to be one of those women for whom pregnancy is a nightmarish succession of health problems, made tolerable only by the prospect of a birth at the end of the ordeal. Ensuring that you are in optimal health, mentally, emotionally, and physically before you conceive will reduce the likelihood of developing annoying health problems during your pregnancy. Likewise, regular exercise is advisable, as is special attention to diet and your increased nutritional requirements. Eating sensibly is just about the biggest investment you can make in the future health of your unborn baby. Poor diet at this time greatly increases the likelihood of giving birth to a stillborn or premature baby. It also makes you more likely to have a difficult birth, with postnatal hemorrhage, and uterine and breast infections. If you eat well while you grow your new baby, both of you will have a happy future of good health to look forward to.

Diet and Pregnancy

"Eating for two" should be your maxim during these months of pregnancy—not when it comes to your calorie intake (which requires eating for one and a quarter), but when it comes to your nutritional requirements. The research evidence proving the value of optimal nutrition before conception and during pregnancy is limitless, much of it dating back as far as the 1930s. Optimal nutrition in the early months will greatly reduce your chances of miscarrying during the high-risk first trimester. Laboratory experiments with rats show that those animals that were fed a diet containing vitamin C and folic acid levels five times higher than the RDA had far fewer miscarriages and produced larger litters of offspring who were also bigger than average. Interestingly, these experiments show that poor nutrient levels which seemingly had no ill effects on the mother produced dire consequences for the offspring. In other words *you* may stay well on a suboptimum diet during your pregnancy, but your unborn child may pay the price. The heavier your baby is at birth, the less risk there is of neonatal health problems, and so one of your aims is to produce a good weight baby. The way to do this? Once again, it's simple—pay attention to your nutrition.

There are other good reasons for eating wisely. Good nutrition during your pregnancy can virtually eliminate your baby's chances of being born with a major birth defect such as spina bifida. Not only will your baby be more likely to be born healthy, it will probably also be born with a potential for intellectual, physical, and emotional development well above the norm. Of course, eating well also pays off for you directly in terms of your own health. You will be much less likely to encounter serious problems that could jeopardize your pregnancy, such as hypertension, edema, preeclampsia, and toxemia.

Being pregnant is a daunting responsibility, and one of your main responsibilities is to ensure that your growing child receives the very best in terms of nutrition. During this time try to make every mouthful a nutritious one, and steer away from any food that contains lots of calories but only limited nutritional value; for instance, cakes, candy, cookies, and other junk foods.

During your pregnancy you will need more:

- Protein
- Calcium
- Iron
- Vitamin E
- Folic acid
- Zinc
- B Complex.

Putting on Weight During Pregnancy

If you eat healthy foods and exercise regularly, you won't have to worry about keeping an eye on the scale. Your grandmother might have been sternly warned about the dangers of gaining too much weight during pregnancy, but thankfully medical thinking in this area has changed. Today, women are told that even if they gain around 28 to 40 pounds during pregnancy, they needn't worry as long as they are eating a nutritious and balanced diet. If you are overweight when you conceive, do not try to lose weight during your pregnancy. Dieting restricts your intake of nutrients essential to your fetus. Research also indicates that dieting at this time causes a metabolic disturbance that can impair the development of your baby's brain and nerves. While you are pregnant your RDA of extra energy is about 300 calories, the aim being to gain at least 15 pounds (and most probably double this) during your pregnancy. Heavier babies are babies with larger and more mature vital organs, which are more prepared to function efficiently after birth.

Protein Requirements During Pregnancy

During pregnancy your nutritional requirements skyrocket. This increased requirement applies to your protein intake, too. Protein is essential for the formation of a healthy placenta, and to build your baby's brain and tissues. Your protein requirements increase from around 45 g to 75 g a day. Your extra requirements can be met by adding more low-fat dairy products (two cups of yogurt or one cup of cottage cheese), low-fat animal proteins (4 ounces of fish and chicken), or vegetarian proteins such as nuts, seeds, tofu, and beans.

Inadequate protein intake at this time also greatly increases your chances of developing the potentially serious problem of toxemia. Studies indicate that in women who take less than 55 g of protein a day, almost one in two will develop some signs of toxemia during pregnancy. On the other hand, women consuming 75 g or more of protein daily showed no signs of this imbalance. The type of extra protein you load up on seems to be important. Animal proteins and full-fat dairy products supply large amounts of cholesterol and saturated fat along with their protein. While most people know that saturated fats are detrimental to their heart and blood vessels, not everyone is aware that these same fats can increase their likelihood of developing toxemia during pregnancy. That's why low-fat animal proteins, such as fish and chicken, and vegetarian proteins are especially indicated.

To ensure that you obtain a complete protein (that is, a protein that supplies all the amino acids needed by your body) from vegetarian sources, certain types of foods must be eaten together.

- Legumes (soybeans, lima beans, navy beans, pinto beans, kidney beans, chick peas, black-eyed beans, and peanuts) should be combined with:

    Barley

    Corn

    Oats

    Rice

    Sesame seeds

    Wheat.

- Rice should be combined with:
    Legumes
    Sesame seeds
    Wheat.
- Wheat should be combined with:
    Legumes
    Rice and soybeans
    Soybeans and peanuts
    Soybeans and sesame seeds.

Calcium

When you are pregnant, your body needs 50 percent more calcium than usual to ensure the proper development of your baby's skeleton. If this extra calcium need isn't met by your diet, your body steals from its own reserves, by leaching the required calcium from your bones. Two or three "calcium deficit" pregnancies could see you well on your way to developing osteoporosis in later life. Osteoporosis has been given much publicity recently because of its crippling consequences. Although this bone-thinning disorder doesn't usually come to light until you are well past your menopause, its insidious beginnings often trace back to your pregnancies and subsequent breastfeeding. Try to aim for an intake of about 1500 mg of calcium per day during pregnancy and breastfeeding. This can be supplied through dairy products, almonds, broccoli, bony fish (such as salmon, herring, sardines), soybeans, tofu, sesame seeds, and tahini.

There are other good and more immediate reasons for being calcium-wise during pregnancy. It is proven to be one of the main preventatives against potentially fatal high blood pressure and eclampsia.

Your Body Needs Iron, Too

During the initial months of pregnancy your body manufactures a huge amount of extra blood, increasing your blood by one-third, and to do this it needs greatly increased supplies of iron. This is why some doctors routinely dish out iron supplements to their pregnant patients. The inorganic ferrous sulphate supplements which are usually administered are the cause of trying times in the bathroom, as they cause terrible constipation. There are good alternatives, such as iron chelate or orotate, which will prevent iron deficiency anemia without causing constipation. Read the section on iron in Chapter 2 for hints on how to maximize your dietary iron. If you are lacking in iron during your pregnancy, the chances are your baby will also be lacking in this crucial mineral. If this is so, he or she will be at a distinct intellectual disadvantage. Infants, toddlers, and school children with low iron levels do not do as well intellectually as their iron-rich peers—something worth thinking about in these days of ever-increasing intellectual and educational demands.

B Complex Vitamins

When you become pregnant your need for B complex vitamins, and in particular B6 and folic acid, increases dramatically. Many of the discomforts associated with pregnancy, such as morning sickness, fluid retention, hemorrhoids, and cramps, can be avoided by ensuring adequate intake of B6. This vitamin is also an important factor in the prevention (and treatment) of toxemia in pregnancy.

Taking B6 supplements in isolation is not a good idea because of the synergistic nature of all the B vitamins. Any one of them taken in isolation can cause deficiencies of other B vitamins. Look first and foremost at supplying large amounts of the B vitamins through your food. Include generous amounts of leafy green vegetables, whole grains, wheat germ, brewer's yeast, and organ meats such as chicken and beef livers (see the chart on p. 60).

A high potency, balanced B complex supplement will provide the extra B6 needed to treat problems such as morning sickness or fluid retention. If you are eating plenty of green leafy vegetables and brewer's yeast and taking your B supplement, you won't have to worry about getting adequate folic acid supplies. Education about this B vitamin should be compulsory for every pregnant woman, because of its proven ability to reduce the likelihood of giving birth to a deformed or handicapped baby (see Chapter 2, pp. 40-41). Lack of this vitamin during pregnancy causes a type of anemia that will not respond to iron supplements. It also predisposes you to hemorrhage during the birth, and increases your chances of premature birth.

During pregnancy your nutrient requirements in general increase. However, your requirement for the B vitamin folacin increases by 100 percent. Not surprisingly, deficiency of this vitamin during pregnancy is extremely common.

Folacin is *the* vitamin to prevent the development of neural tube defect (spina bifida) in your fetus. This common defect affects around 2 in every 100 live births, and causes malformation of the brain and spinal cord. Ensure that your intake of folacin is at least 800 mcg a day by eating plenty of green vegetables and fresh fruit and by using a multi-B complex supplement throughout your pregnancy.

Vitamin E

You need more than twice the normal amount of vitamin E when you are pregnant. Wheat germ and cold-pressed wheat germ oil are two extremely important sources of this vitamin. If you are using an inorganic iron tonic, your absorption of this vitamin will be hindered. Take iron and vitamin E supplements at least eight hours apart.

Vegetarians in Pregnancy

If you are a vegetarian, you should pay particular attention to your zinc intake before and during your pregnancy. Vegetarians are often lacking in zinc because one of the most reliable dietary sources of this mineral is red meat. Zinc is one of those nutrients you need in an ongoing, regular supply, as you are unable to stockpile reserves. Low zinc supplies mean a higher incidence of low birth weight babies with postnatal health problems. This nutrient is also essential for normal cell division such as occurs during pregnancy, and zinc deficiency hinders the speed and normality of this process. It also increases your likelihood of maternal health problems such as hypertension, preeclampsia, and toxemia.

If you are taking iron or folacin supplements during your pregnancy, be aware that these nutrients compete with zinc for absorption—the more of these vitamins you absorb, the less zinc you absorb. Combat this by making sure your supplement (or an additional supplement) also contains between 10 and 30 mg of zinc.

Other Nutrients

During your pregnancy you also need more vitamins A and C, and the trace mineral iodine. If you follow the healthy eating outline in Chapter 2, paying particular attention to foods containing calcium, iron, B vitamins, C, and A, you can rest assured you are giving your baby the best start in life.

Things To "Have Not" During Pregnancy

While you can choose whether to have a drink or smoke a cigarette, your unborn child cannot. If you drink, so does he or she. If you have a cigarette, so too does your baby. As pregnancy is such a short time span, and the detrimental effects of smoking, drinking, and drug-taking during pregnancy have been so clearly demonstrated, use a little willpower and simply *don't indulge!*

Smoking

Smoking affects your baby in a whole range of undesirable ways. Your baby is more likely to be stillborn, or at least come into the world prematurely. A study at the Royal Hospital for Women in Sydney, Australia, showed that 21 percent of mothers who smoke had miscarried at least once before, compared with only 16 percent of non-smoking mothers.

Non-smoking mothers had a stillbirth incidence of 12 in every 1000 births, but in mothers who smoked more than 10 cigarettes a day the rate rose alarmingly to 21 per 1000 births. Even if your baby does last the full term, he or she will probably be of low birth weight, and with a smaller head and chest than the baby of a non-smoking mother. Every cigarette you smoke during pregnancy causes fetal distress as shown by an abnormal fetal heart rate. If you smoke just one cigarette, your baby's heartbeat will change suddenly and dramatically. It may increase by up to 39 beats a minute, or decrease by up to 17 beats a minute.

Caffeine

Even a simple pleasure like a cup of brewed coffee can be a risk to your unborn baby, if indulged in excessively. A recent study using a sample group of 800 women in Utah found that there was a high incidence of problems during pregnancy with high miscarriage and stillbirth rates among women drinking more than seven cups of coffee a day. Fetuses and newborns metabolize caffeine differently than do adults. While adult livers rapidly break down the caffeine from a cup of coffee, the unborn or newborn child seems to be unable to perform this detoxification function with ingested caffeine. Up to 83 percent of the caffeine they ingest is passed out of their body in their urine unchanged. Compare this to the one percent incidence of unchanged caffeine excreted by a fully grown adult!

What Happens to Your Body During Pregnancy

Although pregnancy is a completely natural condition, it is nonetheless a time of great physical and emotional change—a change that can be stressful if your body is ill prepared for it. By the twelfth week of pregnancy your production of blood will increase to meet your increased blood volume requirement. Your heart will pump more quickly to move this increased load of blood. Many of your organs will have an increased supply of blood, in particular your uterus, with a 150 percent increase in blood supply. If you are physically fit and exercise regularly before your baby is conceived, your body is much better prepared to cope with this increased load on your cardiovascular system.

Another good reason for being at your peak of fitness when you conceive is the changes to your respiratory system which will occur as your uterus grows larger. In the latter part of pregnancy your hugely swollen uterus actually pushes up against your diaphragm, reducing the expansion of your lungs when you breathe. Your hormones also increase your sensitivity to carbon dioxide, which in turn causes you to tire easily during exercise. In a physically fit body these changes are less noticeable.

Obviously your body undergoes enormous hormonal changes at this time. Among other things, these changed hormonal balances soften your connective tissue and loosen your joints and ligaments, greatly increasing your risk of injury through unwise exercise. During pregnancy it is a good idea to perform lots of limbering and stretching exercises, and as much as possible to avoid jarring, high-impact-type exercise.

As your uterus enlarges it literally pushes your other abdominal organs (such as your stomach and digestive tract) out of the way. This may cause nausea or heartburn throughout the latter stages of your pregnancy. The lower part of your uterus expands downwards, pressing on your vagina and the strong band of muscle called the pelvic floor, this cradle of muscle is responsible for supporting your pelvic organs such as the uterus, bladder, and intestines. Unless it is exercised like the rest of your body, the pelvic floor can become weak and ineffective (see Chapter 3, pp. 78–79 for information on pelvic floor exercises).

What Sort of Exercise for Pregnancy?

If you are very fit before you become pregnant, and are used to regular and vigorous exercise, there is no reason why you should not continue a regular (but probably somewhat modified) exercise regime. If you are unfit when you conceive, it is generally considered inadvisable to embark suddenly on a rigorous aerobic workout regime at this time. By all means begin to exercise with gentle workouts such as swimming, brisk walking, and stretching exercises. Do not suddenly decide, however, when you are 10 weeks pregnant that now is the time to take out a gym membership and go to three aerobics classes a week.

Pregnancy can be enjoyed more fully if you are fit and healthy when you conceive. There are benefits to exercising before and during your pregnancy. You will probably experience less physical discomfort in the way of backaches, constipation, and varicose veins. Your balance, coordination, and appearance will be better, and your pre-pregnancy shape will probably be a lot easier to regain after the birth. Exercise will also improve your circulation and respiration and give you a lot more energy for coping with the physical and emotional changes occurring in your body.

There are a few general "don'ts" when it comes to exercising during pregnancy:

- Try to avoid high-impact exercise such as aerobics and jogging, as in pregnancy the general loosening of connective tissue and joints increases your probability of injury.

- Try to avoid exercising to the point of becoming overheated. Prolonged periods of exercise that increase your temperature dramatically can have a marked detrimental effect on your unborn child.

Help for Minor Health Problems of Pregnancy

Morning Sickness

This has to be one of the most common, and in some cases the most incapacitating, of the problems encountered during pregnancy. Well-meaning people telling you that it will wear off by the fourteenth or fifteenth week are of no use to you if you are spending half of every day with your head down the toilet! The term "morning sickness" is a bit of a misnomer, as it can last all day, or occur in the evening, or at meal times, rather than in the morning. While the exact cause of morning sickness is still not known, it seems that this phenomenon of pregnancy can be interpreted as a positive signal that all is as it should be with your hormones.

Women who have morning sickness have lower incidences of premature birth, stillbirth, and miscarriages. This doesn't mean that you have to passively put up with the nausea and vomiting. There are some drug-free, safe solutions for you to try. No matter how sick you are, unless your doctor advises, don't use drugs to help you over this hurdle. The cost to your developing baby can be very great.

The simplest, and in some cases the only, therapy you need is a dietary change. You may well find that by paying attention to the frequency and type of meals you eat, your sickness can be kept under control. Always start the day with a warm drink and a little dry toast or crackers *before* you get out of bed. From there on, eat small amounts frequently, rather than sticking to the usual three large meals a day routine. Keep plenty of high-protein foods around (such as nuts, seeds, low-fat dairy products, cold chicken) for snacking on. Fatty foods, refined carbohydrates, sugar, and acid foods can all worsen your nausea. Last thing at night have a high-protein snack, which will digest slowly during the night. Try to avoid coffee, as it causes your stomach to release a lot of acid, which in turn can worsen your nausea. There are a variety of pleasant and therapeutic herbal teas that you can experiment with instead. Peppermint tea settles the stomach and helps with the feelings of nausea. Chamomile and spearmint teas are also useful for this. Try making a cup of spearmint tea and adding a half teaspoon of powdered ginger and a little honey to taste. Ginger is very effective for all types of sickness and many sailors swear it keeps seasickness at bay. The Chinese suggest rubbing the tongue with a slice of fresh ginger whenever you feel nauseous.

Vitamin B6 May Help

If you still feel sick despite all the dietary changes, vitamin B_6 may offer you a solution. This vitamin has been used for years to treat the nausea of pregnancy, seasickness, and nausea resulting from chemotherrapy. Your B6 should be taken as part of a balanced B complex, rather than on its own. It should be taken with meals, in split doses through the day. The required dosage varies from as low as 30 mg a day, up to 600 mg a day. Don't take more than 100 mg a day of this vitamin without professional supervision.

Acupuncture

Acupuncture has been used for thousands of years in China to treat morning sickness. During pregnancy your energy, or chi, changes dramatically. Morning sickness is usually associated with an excess of liver energy and a deficiency of stomach and spleen energy. By using acupuncture to cool the "rebellious" chi of the liver and strengthen the digestive organs, morning sickness can be lessened or completely prevented. Traditionally, one of the most effective acupuncture points for any type of nausea is a point on the underside of the forearm, about two thumb widths above the wrist crease, between the two tendons. Most drugstores sell "sea bands," which you wear around your arm, to exert constant pressure on this point. By stimulating this acupuncture point, the band helps to lessen the severity of your nausea. Of course sea bands can also be used to cope with morning sickness.

Homeopathy for Morning Sickness

- *Tabacum.* For nausea with no vomiting, and if you have a pale complexion, feel very cold, and salivate profusely.

- *Petroleum.* For nausea with or without vomiting, and if you have diarrhea and profuse sweating; a hearty appetite despite the nausea, and the appetite is good again straight after vomiting.

- *Ipecac.* For severe vomiting when you cannot keep any food down and if there is constant, severe nausea and excessive salivation, no thirst, and you suffer emotional irritability.

- *Phosphorus.* If you have a thirst for cold water, but vomit the moment it becomes warm.

- *Nux Vomica.* Useful for irritability and short temper and if you retch each morning and are bad-tempered until midday. This type of vomiting occurs in a sudden spasm, following breakfast. Vomit tastes bitter and acidic.

- *Natrum Phos* (sodium phosphate). For nausea without any other symptoms.

- *Pulsatilla.* For fair-haired (and often blue-eyed) exceptionally sensitive women who are emotional and tearful. You may feel insecure, with rapidly changing moods. This type of nausea comes and goes but is most prevalent in the late afternoon or evening. There is no thirst and the tongue may be covered with a thick, whitish-yellow coating.

- *Sepia.* For exhaustion and fatigue and often low-down, dragging abdominal pains. Despite feeling sick, the appetite remains good, and is often excessive. The vomit is pale and may contain mucus.

Heartburn

Usually, morning sickness has passed by the sixteenth week of pregnancy. The other common digestive disorder which may be troublesome tends to occur in the last 12 weeks of pregnancy. The first time you have heartburn you may imagine yourself to be having a heart attack. The pain can be quite intense, but has nothing to do with a heart problem. Heartburn is caused by acid from your stomach rising up into the esophagus (the tube that connects your mouth to your stomach). Help yourself by avoiding spicy foods, coffee, and alcohol, and try not to eat a large evening meal before going to bed. Sipping cold chamomile tea may also help.

Try to avoid excessive use of pharmaceutical antacids such as bicarbonate of soda, as the sodium they contain can cause fluid retention and swelling. Titralac tablets interfere with your absorption and utilization of iron, a crucial mineral which many pregnant women fail to get adequate supplies of anyway.

Homeopathy can help you deal with this problem safely. Capsicum or Natrum Phos in a 3 c potency can be taken whenever you experience your heartburn. Alternatively, chew on a couple of sodium phosphate tablets whenever you feel an attack coming on.

Constipation and Hemorrhoids

In preparation for birth, the hormone progesterone relaxes all the ligaments and smooth muscles in your body, including the muscles that make up the walls of the large intestine and colon. Consequently, many hours may be spent reading the newspaper on the toilet, waiting for the elusive bowel movement to happen! Try to counteract the problem of constipation by including plenty of fiber in your diet—eat plenty of raw vegetables and fruit, and drink at least eight glasses of water a day.

Linseed has a gentle laxative effect. It is non-addictive and does not cause griping. Soak two tablespoons of whole linseed overnight and sprinkle this on your food during the day. A glass of freshly squeezed lemon juice and hot water before breakfast may help "jump start" a lazy bowel.

Make sure you keep up your regular exercise to stimulate the intestines to contract, and to prevent constipation. Constantly straining to have a bowel movement will hasten the development of hemorrhoids (commonly called piles). Piles are actually varicose veins on the edge of the anus. They may occur up inside the rectum or protrude outside the body. Piles cause anal itching and burning, and sometimes also bleed. It is very common for trouble with piles to date back to the time of your first pregnancy, when constipation and straining in the toilet may have been a problem for several months. You can avoid or minimize trouble with piles by following the guidelines to avoid constipation. Soft, bulky stools that are passed without straining will prevent piles. Don't spend "time out" relaxing on the toilet with a newspaper, as long periods of time spent sitting in this position encourage the prolapse of your rectal veins, and the formation of piles.

Certain nutritional deficiencies will predispose you to getting piles. Vitamin C and bioflavinoids are essential to keep the walls of your blood vessels strong. When these nutrients are lacking, your capillaries and veins weaken and become more prone to prolapse and ballooning, causing piles and varicose veins. Besides using a vitamin C and bioflavinoid supplement, you can increase your dietary intake by eating plenty of fruits and raw vegetables. The pith of citrus fruit, and plums, apricots, and grapes supply large amounts of bioflavinoids. Try making a buckwheat cereal for breakfast, or adding buckwheat flour to your whole grain flour when baking. This grain is one of the richest dietary sources of bioflavinoids.

Herbal and Homeopathic Remedies

If you already have hemorrhoids and the pain is driving you mad, there are some simple, effective remedies to be found in your health shop. A bottle of witch hazel lotion is a cheap and useful way to deal with your troubles. Soak a cotton pad with this astringent lotion and bathe your hemorrhoids several times a day. This stops itching and pain, and shrinks the hemorrhoids. The herb pilewort has been used for centuries for this problem, and today is the main ingredient in herbal hemorrhoidal ointment.

Several homeopathic remedies are useful for dealing with hemorrhoids if you do develop them despite your best intentions. Aesculus is useful for those external piles that look like a small bunch of purple grapes. The rectum burns and there may be sharp shooting pains up through the rectum. Nitric acid treats piles that feel like needles or splinters in the rectum, while Nux Vomica is appropriate for piles that are characterized by constant, maddening itching, which is relieved by cool baths. Sulphur also treats itching piles, but these piles are made worse by bathing, rubbing, or standing. Arnica is useful for piles that develop following birth, usually as a result of bearing down during the birth.

Varicose Veins

Varicose veins which appear for the first time during pregnancy can cause your legs to ache and your ankles to swell, or they may do no more that look unsightly and cause mental anguish. The same hormones that cause the muscles of the bowel to become lax cause the walls of the blood vessels to soften and distend. The veins in the legs contain tiny, one-way valves which help the movement of blood back up out of the legs and toward the heart. When these valves become weakened or softened (as often happens during pregnancy), the blood tends to pool more in the leg veins. The blood in the arteries is pumped around the body by the never-ending action of the heart. Blood flowing in the veins is under much less pressure than arterial blood. Regular exercise helps to stimulate blood flow in the veins and is consequently one of the most effective ways to prevent varicose veins.

In the latter stage of pregnancy, the very size and weight of the fetus can obstruct the blood vessels at the top of the legs and prevent adequate return of blood from the legs, causing varicose veins to worsen. So, if you want to try to avoid these unsightly, snake-like blemishes, make sure that you invest in a good pair of walking shoes, and put them to good use every day. Never sit for long periods of time without flexing calf muscles or getting up for a quick walk. When you are sitting, put your feet up whenever possible, and never sit with your ankles or legs crossed. If your veins are really bad, you may be wise to wear support hose. Constipation and an overloaded bowel can actually cause pressure, which restricts blood return from the legs—another good reason to keep up your "rabbit food" and exercise regime. You can use witch hazel compresses on your vericose veins as well as your piles.

Varicose veins are indicative of weak blood vessel walls (the same as piles), and consequently, attention to ensuring plentiful nutrients needed to strengthen these blood vessels will help you with your problem. These nutrients include vitamin E, vitamin C, and the bioflavinoids, in particular rutin. As well as including plenty of food sources of these nutrients, a rutin supplement in the region of 200 mg a day is advisable.

The common garden daisy provides one of the homeopathic remedies useful for varicose veins—Bellis Perennis is useful for varicose veins which ache or throb and feel worse with any kind of touch or with heat, but better during exercise or cold applications. Witch hazel is the raw material used for the homeopathic remedy Hamamelis, which is useful for relieving the pain of varicose veins.

Leg Cramps

Anyone who has ever woken up in the dead of night feeling the excruciating, vice-like pain of leg cramps will want to do everything possible to counteract the increased tendency to this problem during pregnancy. Cramps at any time usually indicate a need for more minerals, in particular calcium and magnesium. This is largely the reason why cramps are especially common in pregnant women, who frequently are not obtaining enough of these minerals to meet their increased requirements. Vitamin

B$_6$ deficiency also causes cramping, and as you have already seen, this is another only too common deficiency in pregnancy. Take your balanced multi-mineral supplement and eat plenty of calcium-rich foods and you will probably never have to cope with this painful problem.

Stretch Marks

Nature is sometimes very unfair. Why is it that your pregnancy, which resulted in a 6-pound baby, left your abdomen looking like a battlefield, while your friend, the mother of a 9-pound newborn, it totally unblemished? The sad fact is, no one can answer your question with certainty. This common scenario seems to refute the theory that gaining too much weight causes stretch marks. Even the tiniest of pregnant tummies can sometimes be prone to stretch marks. So what can you do to lessen your risk?

Starting from the first trimester, make a brisk abdominal massage a part of your daily routine. Do it for yourself, or include your partner in the fun. Use a light oil such as cold-pressed almond oil or apricot oil. If you don't mind the messy yellow stains that it can leave, wheat germ oil is especially useful because of its high vitamin E content. Remember to massage your hips and breasts as well, because these parts stretch a lot too!

If you do develop stretch marks despite your best efforts, vitamin E can help minimize your long-term scarring. Pierce a couple of 500 iu of vitamin E capsules each day and rub the oil into the marks. Persevere for several months, because this treatment doesn't work overnight but your efforts should show a marked improvement.

There is a theory that stretch marks occur more in women who are zinc-deficient. This hasn't been conclusively proven, but it would benefit you and your baby to make sure that your zinc intake is high throughout your pregnancy (see Chapter 7).

American nutritionist Paavo Airola recommends that pregnant women use his "formula S," applied topically to the abdomen, breasts, and thighs daily. This concoction consists of a base of four tablespoons of cold-pressed olive oil to which is added 4000 iu of mixed tocopherol vitamin E and 50,000 iu of vitamin A. Once mixed, the formula needs to be refrigerated and kept in an air-tight container to prevent rancidity.

Toxemia

Toxemia, or preeclampsia, is one of the most serious and sometimes life-threatening problems that you can encounter during your pregnancy. The warning signs of toxemia are high blood pressure, fluid retention, and protein showing in your urine sample. With today's nutritional knowledge, no woman need ever develop it. Toxemia rarely develops in women with sound nutrition and adequate protein intake. Make sure that your protein intake is high, drink plenty of water, and follow your tastebuds when it comes to salt intake. Toxemia is a dietary deficiency illness; in particular, it is the result of inadequate dietary protein. If you do develop toxemia, there are other nutritional supplements you will need to take. Because this condition is potentially very serious, consult a nutritionally trained health professional rather than self-prescribing.

Vitamin B6, magnesium, and calcium have all proven to be effective as part of the management of toxemia. B6 is nature's diuretic, and will assist in easing fluid retention and lowering your blood pressure. It works best when taken along with magnesium. You may be worrying that increasing your salt intake will only serve to further increase your already high blood pressure. It's true that for many years the immediate response to high blood pressure in pregnant women (or anybody else) was to advise an immediate and total withdrawal of salt from the diet. Ironically, there is now a reliable body of evidence which shows that eliminating salt actually makes matters worse by resulting in a further increase in blood pressure. When you cut out salt, your body releases a hormone that triggers a series of biochemical events, culminating in your blood vessels constricting and thus actually increasing your blood pressure. If your blood pressure is high during pregnancy, pay attention to what your tastebuds are telling you and make salt a part of your daily diet.

Miscarriage

Many women in the reproductive years miscarry without ever knowing that they were pregnant. A late period that is particularly clotty and heavy may be a miscarriage which passes with little more than a few menstrual cramps. However, miscarriage can be an emotionally devastating loss for women who know they are pregnant and are happy about their condition.

Miscarrying at eight weeks of pregnancy has as much of an emotional impact as miscarrying at 16 or 20 weeks. Many women feel a fetus is a baby, no matter how developed it is. The impact of early miscarriage is greatly underestimated in society. While most people commiserate and support the couple who give birth to a dead child, or whose infant dies soon after birth, there is often little empathy or understanding for the loss of a baby in the early weeks or months of pregnancy. Women are told that they will get "over it," and should "try again" soon. Or else, your loss may be private, with few if any friends even knowing you were pregnant—again denying you the opportunity of emotional support.

Miscarriage is common, with 10 percent of all pregnancies ending this way—more if you include those miscarriages that were thought to be simply late periods. A miscarriage, or spontaneous abortion (the technical term), is said to have occurred if you lose your baby before 28 weeks of pregnancy. After this your loss is referred to as a stillbirth.

Despite miscarriage being such a common occurrence, very little is really known about what causes it in many cases. Only about 60 percent of fetuses that miscarry are found to have some kind of chromosomal abnormality. That leaves 40 percent of miscarriages with no perceivable fetal abnormality. Other possible causes of miscarriage include maternal hormonal abnormalities; endocrine imbalances such as hypothyroidism and diabetes; uterine abnormalities including fibroids, incompetent cervix, or malpositioning of the uterus; infections; and accidents. Smoking, drinking alcohol, and high levels of stress are also high-risk factors for miscarriage.

One of the major causes of miscarriage is an insufficiency of hormones at the time of the third month of pregnancy. At this point the woman's production of progesterone (secreted by the corpus luteum) decreases, and the placenta takes over the role of progesterone production. If the placenta fails to secrete adequate levels of this hormone, the pregnancy is terminated and results in a miscarriage.

One of the less acknowledged, but crucial, factors in triggering miscarriage is poor maternal nutrition. Miscarriages are also more likely if you have had one before, if you took more than six months to conceive, and if you are over 35 years of age.

If you are pregnant, there are certain obvious precautions you can take to decrease your likelihood of miscarriage. These include total abstinence from alcohol and cigarettes, reducing exposure to stress as much as possible, and paying careful attention to your diet and nutritional status.

Nutritional Supplements To Guard Against Miscarriage

Following the nutritional advice for a healthy pregnancy discussed earlier in this chapter is a good place to start. However, when it comes to guarding against miscarriage, certain nutrients play a particularly important role. These include the B vitamins (especially B_6), zinc, vitamin C and bioflavionoids, and vitamin E.

During the first three or four months of pregnancy, your body's increased output of progesterone is vital for the viability of your pregnancy. Low progesterone production at this time can result in miscarriage, and it has been discovered that a B_6 deficiency can indirectly lead to this low output of hormone. Whenever the concentration of estrogen in your bloodstream increases, there is a reflex reduction in your production of progesterone. Vitamin B_6 is one of the vital nutrients that allows your liver to convert your circulating estrogen into a water-soluble form which can easily be passed via your urine from the body. Without adequate supplies of this nutrient, the estrogen levels build up and up, and in turn your production of progesterone is decreased—and if it falls low enough, there may be insufficient quantity to maintain your growing fetus.

Once again the importance of zinc becomes apparent. This trace element is vital for the normal development of your fetus. Low-zinc diets result in a higher incidence of miscarriage, and this is partly due to the fact that adequate zinc is required to allow your body to absorb the crucial pregnancy nutrient, folic acid. Zinc also enhances the absorption and functioning of B_6.

When an egg is fertilized and makes its way to the uterus to implant, the endometrium (lining of the uterus) provides a thick, lush, nutrient-rich groundsoil in which to grow. This lining is extraordinarily richly supplied with blood, flowing through a complex network of tiny blood vessels. For the egg to implant and develop into a fetus, this thick lining of blood vessels must be strong and resilient, and two of the nutrients most involved with keeping it this way are vitamin C and bioflavinoids. In terms of your diet, plenty of fresh vegetables will ensure an adequate intake of these nutrients. If you have a history of miscarriage, the scientific research shows that it would be very much worth your while to use vitamin C and bioflavinoid supplements right from the start of your pregnancy.

No look at any aspect of human sexual functioning would be complete without mention of the benefits of vitamin E. This oil-soluble vitamin is particularly lacking in most Western diets, and is crucial for reproductive functioning and carrying your baby to full term. Vitamin E is essential for the fertilized egg to embed itself firmly into the endometrium, and for the placenta to develop around it. Using vitamin E supplements can safely be part of your pre-conceptual program for achieving optimum reproductive health, and continuing to use it (in doses of 300 to 400 iu daily) during the first three or four months of your pregnancy will help safeguard you against the risk of miscarriage.

Homeopathic help

If you experience any of the symptoms of threatened miscarriage, then your first course of action must be to contact your doctor immediately. However, you can also help yourself at the same time by using an indicated homeopathic remedy.

- *Arnica*. This is a first-line-of-action remedy, especially if you have lost a lot of blood or are in any kind of shock (physical or emotional).

- *Belladonna*. The blood lost is bright red and accompanied by severe contractions of the uterus. The vagina and lower abdominal area become extremely sensitive to any kind of touch or movement. There is often severe lower back pain with a general feeling of dragging down pressure.

- *Secale*. The blood loss is dark, blackish, and smelly, and may be accompanied by diarrhea.

- *Sabina*. Severe, painful contractions of the uterus result in loss of bright red blood mixed with darkish clots. You seek fresh air and cannot stand heat.

Chapter 9

Birth Pain—
The Natural Approach

Most first-time mothers anticipate the birth of their baby with a heady mixture of excitement and fear. Besides anxiously hoping that their baby will be born normal and healthy, the most common fear can be summed up in one word—*pain*. "What will the pain feel like?"; "Will I be able to cope with it?"; "Will I have to use some sort of pain relief?"

These are all normal anxieties. The modern hospital birth bears little resemblance to the childbirth experiences of previous centuries, or even decades. Today's drugs make it possible to have a baby and experience no more pain than during a menstrual period. However, the pharmacological pain relievers such as gas, pethidine, and epidurals are not without their drawbacks.

Gas, Pethidine, and Epidurals

Gas, which is a mixture of laughing gas (nitrous oxide) and oxygen, is the most common and acceptable form of orthodox pain relief. You administer this to yourself, as and when you need it, breathing it in at the start of a contraction. Gas can be quite effective to take the edge off your pain, and because it passes out of your body between contractions, it doesn't pass into your baby's body in large amounts.

As soon as your baby is born and begins to breathe, the traces of gas disappear from his or her blood very quickly. Unfortunately, some women find gas useless, and complain of dizziness. An injection of pethidine is often the next step up if gas isn't effective. Ideally, this will ease your pain and induce a state of relaxation. Commonly, though, it can leave you feeling nauseous and "spaced out" or slightly drunk. Pethidine quickly crosses the placenta and affects your baby. "Pethidine babies" tend to be drowsier and floppier at birth and are often slower to suck the nipple.

The modern birth painkiller supreme is the epidural. It is the only labor painkiller that can completely remove *all* pain, and in fact all feeling, from the abdomen down. Administering an epidural (a spinal injection) is a highly skilled process that must be performed by an anesthetist. Although extremely effective as a painkiller, an epidural often signifies an escalation in the technological intervention required for the rest of the birth. Once you have the injection you will be unable to move around, and will be confined to bed. Because you will no longer be able to feel your contractions, you will need to wear an electric belt monitor. Ideally, your epidural is timed to wear off by the second stage of birth so that you can feel your pushing impulses. This is not always successfully judged, and if your epidural hasn't worn off by this stage, your pushing will be dramatically less effective. You simply won't be able to feel what you are doing. If this happens, your chances of needing a forceps delivery are markedly increased.

Although none of these pain-killing drugs are perfect, there are occasions when their relief is warranted and gratefully received. However, more and more American women want to manage their birth pain using a variety of safe and gently non-drug methods. A growing number of women are opting for home births, and the vast majority of these home births occur without any form of drug pain relief, producing healthy babies and happy moms.

Pain and Natural Solutions

Pain is a subjective sensation. Every woman perceives pain differently and has her own unique pain tolerance level. It helps to acknowledge that birth will be painful, but that the pain is a productive and positive pain which will end, and which will be greatly rewarded.

The Western world is conditioned to think of pain of any sort as unnecessary and unacceptable, and to reach for the painkillers quickly. Fear and anxiety can greatly compound the pain of childbirth. Simply being in the unfamiliar surroundings of a hospital can make you tense. Other factors that can increase your sensation of pain include being confined to a bed on your back, because you are wired up to a drip or a monitor. Thankfully, most modern hospitals are now supportive of independent and free movement while you are in labor. Being allowed to listen to your body and to move accordingly allows you to choose the least painful position at any given moment. Artificial speeding up of contractions using a drip or pessary tends to produce stronger and more painful contractions. Emotional support and caring from your birth team can greatly reduce your need for any sort of pain relief.

One of the reasons that home births are increasingly popular is the acknowledgment of the importance of the relationship between the birthing mother and the midwife. Home birth mothers often choose their midwives as soon as they know they are pregnant. This allows many months in which to form a close relationship. There are several meetings with the midwife throughout the pregnancy, and opportunities to discuss your fears, likes, and dislikes so that your midwife knows exactly what kind of birth you are hoping for. Being in the familiar surroundings of home, friends, or family greatly reduces your fear, and in turn your pain. In Holland most births occur at home, unlike the United States, where by far the majority still occur in hospitals. In Holland painkillers are used in only 5 percent of births, compared to 85 percent of births in New Zealand. The statistics speak for themselves.

Tips for Reducing the Pain

Whether you give birth in a hospital or at home, there are several common sense practical steps you can take to reduce your pain, and to make your birthing a happy day to remember.

First, once your contractions begin, stay up and active for as long as possible. While they are not too strong, walk around and lean against a table or a wall during the actual contractions. Staying upright gives you the added assistance of gravity. Upright positions also allow the maximum blood supply to your baby, and reduce the chances of your baby becoming distressed. Lying on your back during labor is the most distressing and painful position possible.

Once your contractions become fiercer and you are unable to walk around, try some more supportive upright positions. Try sitting upright with your legs flopped apart, or squatting or standing leaning across a bed. It will help to have some object such as a lighted candle, a painting, or a flower to focus and concentrate on.

Massage can be wonderfully soothing and distracting when contractions become difficult to manage. Firm, hard massage across the lower back helps with back pain, and gentle fingertip stroking across the abdomen soothes tired muscles. Encourage your partner to practice massage techniques before labor day. A full bladder makes contractions more painful, so remember to empty it frequently!

Homeopathic and Herbal Remedies

Complementary therapies offer many easily administered and safe options for dealing with your birth pain. Cell salts are homeopathic preparations of minerals. When labor begins, a dose of Kali. Phos. (potassium phosphate) every half-hour for a few hours will promote effective labor. Cell salts are available from most health stores and are completely non-toxic.

There are several homeopathic remedies useful during and after labor. The two most commonly used are Caulophyllum and Arnica. Caulophyllum is the homeopathic remedy made from the herb blue cohosh—an herb that was traditionally used to prepare the uterus for childbirth. Taken for three or four weeks before the birth, Caulophyllum tones the uterus and prepares it for the hard work ahead. Caulophyllum 30 c should be taken one dose a week, from weeks 36 to 38, and then one dose daily from weeks 38 to 40.

Homeopathic Arnica (made from "fall herb") stands supreme as a treatment for all types of physical shock, trauma, and pain. Arnica 200 c should be taken twice daily for three days after the birth, to prevent bruising and to aid healing with a minimum of pain. This really is a quite remarkable treatment, which I have used myself and recommended to many women, with impressive results.

Herbal remedies offer another alternative for coping with pain. They can be used during the actual birth, and as a preparation for birth, beginning as early as three months into your pregnancy. After the third month of pregnancy, red raspberry leaf tea can be drunk two to three times daily. Raspberry leaves are rich in iron and as such are a useful supplement to meet your increased iron requirements. This herb is also reputed to prevent hemorrhage and regulate muscle contractions in the uterus during delivery. A recent book on the subject of home birth describes an herbal tea to be drunk for six weeks before the birth to prepare the uterus for the work ahead. The tea is made from equal parts of squawvine, blessed thistle, red raspberry, black cohosh, and pennyroyal. Mix these herbs together in a large container, and make the tea using one teaspoon of this mixture to one cup of boiling water. Drink one cup night and morning.

When you are in labor, you can take herbs in the form of herbal ice cubes. Sucking the ice helps prevent thirst and a dry mouth. In the days before your birth, prepare the ice cubes by making strong infusions of herbal tea and freezing them in ice cube trays. If you are having a hospital birth, you will need to transport your ice in a portable pack! Useful herbs to prepare include blue cohosh; peppermint (helps relieve tension and is a mild painkiller); chamomile (an anti-spasmodic and gentle sedative); valerian (tastes terrible but is a very useful anti-spasmodic and quite a strong sedative); and passionflower, for its calming effects.

"Rescue remedy" is the most commonly used of all the Bach flowers. It is especially useful to calm and relax you if you feel fearful and tense during labor. Simply add five drops to a glass of water and have it on hand to sip as required.

It is proven that nutritionally deficient women tend to have more painful and prolonged labors. The minerals calcium and magnesium are especially important to assist with the effective and coordinated contractions of the uterus muscle. If you are calcium-deficient, the effectiveness of your uterine muscle contractions is reduced, or else you experience contractions that will not stop, causing cramping. This is one very good incentive to ensure that you meet your increased calcium requirements during your pregnancy! Calcium and magnesium supplements can be taken during your labor as well.

Acupuncture

Many home birth midwives, and some doctors, are trained to provide acupuncture for pain relief during birth. Acupuncture during childbirth has a long history, stretching back some 3500 years in China, even though it is a relatively new concept in the West. Acupuncture is not only useful for pain control—it is also effectively used to induce labor, turn breech babies, strengthen contractions, and prevent hemorrhage. It is a highly effective and safe therapy for ante-natal and postnatal problems, as well as for the birth itself. More and more hospitals allow you to have a registered acupuncturist with you during your labor, if your doctor is unable to provide this service.

Finally, try not to form too rigid and dogmatic a picture of what your birth will be like. If you are absolutely determined to have a completely natural birth, you will be very shocked and disappointed if it turns out to be impossible. Don't be disappointed and angry with yourself if you find that you do need to use drugs to cope with your pain. If you are not coping, being a brave martyr will achieve nothing. The most important outcome (whatever help you need to accept) is the birth of a healthy baby to a healthy mother!

Chapter 10

Healing After the Birth

Giving birth may well be one of the most spiritually and physically rewarding experiences of your life. The nine months of waiting and wondering, and putting up with all sorts of discomforts, seem inconsequential when you first hold your newborn. However, from the tremendous emotional high of birth, there may come a rude and sudden crash back to earth as you encounter a whole new set of problems and discomforts to deal with—a bottom which feels as though it has been crushed with a steamroller, sore and itchy stitches, piles, and swollen breasts! What rewards for all your hard work! Added to the physical changes your body continues to go through for some months are the emotional and lifestyle changes your new baby will inevitably bring.

You can minimize your postnatal difficulties by realizing that giving birth is not the ultimate act that signifies the end of the changes of pregnancy. Your body and emotions need to be nurtured and loved in the days and weeks following the birth. Try not to neglect your own needs, as you become absorbed with your wonderful, demanding new dependent. Care for yourself enough to eat properly, drink plenty, sleep, and rest whenever you can, and take up the offers of help from others.

Tearing or Episiotomy?

There is an ongoing debate among professionals involved with the birthing process as to whether an episiotomy (which is a surgical cut through the muscles between your vagina and your anus) or a natural tear is the fastest healing and least traumatic option during childbirth. On the one hand come most of the obstetricians and some GPs who stand firmly in the camp of "episiotomy for all women." On the other side of the argument are some GPs and most of the home birth midwives who claim that tears heal faster and are less painful.

Whichever experience you had, you'll be wanting some relief from your injury. First, you can minimize the degree of bruising and trauma suffered during birth by using the homeopathic remedy Arnica. Arnica 200 c potency can be taken twice daily for three days following the birth. Follow the usual homeopathic protocol, as outlined in Chapter 13. The homeopathic remedy Bellis Perennis 30 c taken as one dose straight after birth will help with pain and any internal injury.

Keep your stitches as clean as possible. Hot baths with a cup of ordinary table salt added will soothe and heal your wound. After each bath, splash the stitches with a little warm water containing calendula lotion. The calendula is very soothing, and greatly decreases healing time. If you can find them, try applying strips of freshly cut papaya to the episiotomy wound. Papaya contains papain, an enzyme that is very soothing and enhances the healing of wounds and burns.

Certain nutrients will hasten you on the road to recovery. Following any kind of surgery (including cesarean and episiotomy) you need more vitamin C, zinc, vitamins A and E, and the B complex. Zinc has been shown to speed the time required for a wound to heal, while vitamin C is crucial for the formation of collagen needed to knit your wound. Vitamins E and C help the formation of new blood vessels at the site of your wound. Vitamin E also helps prevent blood clots. Vitamin E oil can also be applied locally to your perineum, to lessen scar tissue formation. The following are recommended supplements to aid recovery from a cesarean or an episiotomy:

- A broad spectrum B complex plus C supplement supplying 50 mg of the main B vitamins plus 500 mg C. Take two a day.

- A multi-mineral formula, preferably supplying chelated or orotate minerals including calcium, magnesium, zinc, and iron. Take one tablet twice daily between meals.

- Vitamin A or beta-carotene. Take one teaspoon of cod liver oil daily, or a glass or fresh carrot juice.

- Vitamin E. Take 200 iu a day.

Piles or Hemorrhoids

This painful problem has already been discussed in Chapter 8 (see pp. 125-126). The same advice applies for dealing with postnatal piles.

It is worth making sure that pregnancy and birth haven't left you with structural problems that will aggravate hemorrhoids. Pregnancy places a great load on your spine, and osteopathic lesions of the lower back are common at this time. During birth the small tailbone at the very end of the spine (called the coccyx) is pushed back to make room for your baby's head to pass down the birth canal. Sometimes the coccyx fails to return to its normal position, leading to a predisposition to permanent piles. It is always a wise health insurance policy to have a checkup with a registered osteopath once your baby is a couple of weeks old.

Your baby has also undergone an arduous journey to enter the world. Every newborn (except, perhaps, those delivered by cesarean) will have some strain patterns in the skull resulting from the journey down the birth canal. Cranial osteopaths are trained to detect and correct these subtle distortions of the skull, and in doing so prevent the development of a variety of future health problems. In many hospitals, all newborns are routinely treated by a cranial osteopath within a day or so of their birth.

Breast Engorgement

When your baby is two or three days old, the thick colostrum in your breasts will be replaced by milk. At first your breasts may be uncomfortably hard and engorged. Take a hot shower and firmly massage the milk down your breasts toward the nipple. Expressing the milk in this way will temporarily relieve the engorgement, and within a day or two the supply and demand of milk will become more balanced.

If hard-caked breasts remain a problem, try applying a peppermint tea poultice. Make up a very strong brew of peppermint tea. Add enough slippery elm powder to form a paste. Spread onto a piece of gauze and fold over, pinching the edges so as not to lose the paste. Place over the engorged breast and cover with a sheet of plastic to retain the heat. Have the poultice as hot as you can comfortably stand, and replace with a fresh hot poultice every 10 minutes. Repeat three or four times.

A similarly effective poultice can be made from ginger root tea. Make this tea from boiling water poured over several teaspoons of grated fresh ginger.

Sore Nipples

A hungry baby can play havoc with nipples unused to the demands of breastfeeding. During your pregnancy, and after the birth, try to expose your nipples to the sun and air as often as possible. A private spot in the backyard is useful for 10-minute daily sun baths. Don't overdo it. This part of your anatomy is not used to the fierce rays of the sun. Massage your nipples with wheat germ oil to keep them supple and to heal any cracks. There is no need to wash off the oil before feeding the baby. In fact, a little wheat germ oil is often given to newborns by home birth midwives, to correct mild jaundice.

To prevent sore nipples, start breastfeeding for only short periods of time, gradually increasing your baby's time at the breast over a couple of days. When you finish the feed, don't simply pull the baby away from the breast. Remember to break the suction by gently sliding a clean finger into the corner of his or her mouth.

Postnatal Depression

If you become an emotional mess a few days after having your baby, simply accept your see-sawing spirits as a normal part of the "after birth" changes your body goes through. Ninety percent of women experience these postnatal blues, as their hormones plummet to pre-pregnancy levels again.

Allow yourself to cry, and accept the emotional support and nurturing of your partner or someone who is close to you. Plenty of cuddles and maybe massages or foot rubs will help relieve your physical tensions. Get as much rest as possible, and remember to eat wholesome, nutritious food. Make sure that you are eating regularly, as it is only too easy to become so involved in caregiving that you neglect your own nutritional requirements. If you go for long periods without eating, your blood sugar levels will plummet, and this in itself is enough to make you shaky, depressed, and tearful.

If your depression becomes gradually worse, rather than resolving itself in a week or so, you may need a little more help adjusting. Around 20 percent of women develop postnatal depression, which can make life quite unbearable for up to 18 months or more after giving birth. Before you resign yourself to accepting that you are in some way unbalanced, give consideration to some of the simple measures you can take to return yourself to your pre-pregnancy sanity. You must be sick of hearing it by now, but, once again, remember that pregnancy and breastfeeding place a huge nutritional strain on your body. If you haven't been receiving enough nutrients through your diet, you may well end up considerably lacking in a range of mood-elevating nutrients by the time your baby is born. In particular, these include all the B complex vitamins, the amino acids (components of protein) tryptophan and phenylalanine, and the minerals calcium and magnesium.

Start your self-help routine by embarking on a nutritional supplementation regime while also paying close attention to ensuring maximum nutrient supply from your food. You will need to take a high potency B complex supplement supplying 50 mg of all the major B vitamins, twice daily with your meals. A multi-mineral tablet supplying a generous amount of calcium and magnesium as well as zinc and manganese should be taken twice daily, preferably between meals (as minerals are absorbed more effectively with the high concentrations of "resting" stomach acid).

Postnatal depression can make you feel as if you are existing with a permanent case of pre-menstrual tension. You may feel irrationally angry and irritable; tearful and over-emotional; lonely; despondent; and frustrated. Your emotional unhappiness is mirrored by physical symptoms, such as insomnia, despite feeling exhausted, headaches, dizziness, food cravings, and a total disinterest in sex.

In a society populated by mythical superwomen, it is sometimes difficult to acknowledge that you are not coping, and that you need some kind of professional support. If you recognize these symptoms of postnatal depression, don't try to stagger on, putting on a brave face for the world. If your symptoms persist despite following the recommended nutritional program, seek some kind of professional help from a counselor, psychotherapist, or doctor accustomed to dealing with this problem. Don't feel guilty or in any way inferior for not coping. Postnatal depression is a physiological problem caused largely by hormonal and chemical imbalances in your body.

Chapter 11

Breastfeeding

Much research indicates that when it comes to nourishing babies, breast is definitely best. Breast milk is more easily digested than formula milk, and consequently more energy is available for growth. Research still hasn't identified all of the components of breast milk, but it clearly contains the perfect balance of protein, fat, and nutrients for growing babies. Breast milk also offers some degree of protection against infection and disease. The mother's antibodies are passed on to her baby, through the milk. These antibodies provide extra protection for the newborn while his or her own immune system gradually develops. Quite commonly, your whole family may come down with a virus or gastric infection, while your newborn breastfed baby remains perfectly well.

In an American study of 20,000 babies under the age of one year, it was found that there were twice as many infections in the bottle-fed infants as the breastfed. Breastfed babies also suffer dramatically fewer allergies than bottle-fed babies. This is particularly important for babies from families that tend to suffer from allergies, eczema, or asthma.

The following are some of the health benefits for breastfed infants:

- Lower cholesterol levels and less incidence of heart disease (as adults) than bottle-fed babies.
- Less incidence of iron deficiency anemia due to the superior absorption of iron from breast milk.
- Fewer allergic problems due to the protective effect of certain enzymes present in breast milk.
- Markedly lower incidence of gastrointestinal upsets, and bacterial and fungal infections, due to the protective antibodies present in breast milk.
- Healthier teeth and jaws, fewer cavities, and less orthodontal work required than bottle-fed babies.
- Breastfeeding has been proven to be protective against crib death.
- Breastfed babies get ill only half as frequently as bottle-fed babies, and they are three times less likely to be admitted to a hospital.

- Breast milk contains the precursors for your baby to manufacture his or her own choline. This B vitamin is important for normal development and function of the brain.

Breastfeeding is also of benefit to you. Even moments after the birth, breastfeeding helps your body in its gradual return to its pre-pregnant condition. The stimulation of sucking the nipple causes the uterus to contract, making postnatal hemorrhage less likely. Over the weeks following birth, this continued stimulation shrinks your uterus back to its original size. There is also evidence that breastfeeding one or several babies reduces your likelihood of developing breast cancer. Even women who haven't given birth can begin to produce milk (for example, for an adopted baby), given the right assistance, usually from La Leche League.

Still, it is not uncommon for breastfeeding mothers to encounter difficulties some time during the nursing period. Common problems include cracked nipples, too much or too little milk, or breast infections (mastitis). None of these problems should signal the end of breastfeeding, though. During the months leading up to the birth, prepare your nipples for the task ahead! Avoid using soap around the nipple area, as this tends to dry out the skin. Simply wash with clean, warm water. Sunbathing is useful to toughen your nipples. In the last few weeks of pregnancy, stimulate your nipples daily. After your shower or bath, briskly rub your nipples with a coarse towel, and gently pull and roll them between your thumb and index finger. You may be more comfortable using a lubricant such as lanolin or vegetable oil on your nipples. Also, try to express a few drops of the thick colostrum which your breasts will already be producing. By expressing colostrum the milk ducts are opened, and the engorgement when your milk comes in tends to be uncomfortable. (See also the section on sore nipples, which begins on page 140.)

Your Diet and Breastfeeding

If you are going to breastfeed and stay well yourself, you must ensure that your diet is the best. While you are breastfeeding, the needs of your baby take precedence over the needs of your own body. Your body will do everything possible to ensure that your breast milk contains its full complement of nutrients—even if this means robbing your body of essential nutrients. If your diet is poor, you will quickly end up with an exhausted, stressed, and undernourished body which, in time, will be unable to produce adequate milk supplies. Before and during the months of breastfeeding, make sure that every mouthful of food counts. Refined foods, sweet foods, and junk food will pile on the weight without providing much in the way of nutrients. Follow the healthy eating guidelines in Chapter 2.

Traditionally, lactating women were encouraged to consume huge quantities of milk and dairy products to supply adequate calcium. Many women are unable to digest cow's milk products adequately, and pass on undigested milk proteins through their breast milk. This can in turn cause windy babies who drive their mothers mad with screams of colic. Many windy babies improve dramatically when their mothers stop eating dairy products.

Inadequate calcium intake while you are breastfeeding can cause leaching of calcium from your bones and lead to osteoporosis in later years. Include plenty of calcium-rich foods, such as almonds, toasted sesame seeds, bony fish (sardines, herrings, salmon, etc.), tofu, soybeans, dark green leafy vegetables, and yogurt. Because yogurt is a fermented food, it can be tolerated by most people, even if they have a sensitivity to other dairy products. It is also wise to use a balanced calcium and magnesium supplement while you are feeding to ensure that your total calcium intake is 1200 mg a day.

You need an extra 50 mg of protein daily, and about 1000 calories more than usual. Breastfed babies with protein-deficient mothers grow much more slowly, and have stunted brain development.

You might find that adding brewer's yeast, or better still torula yeast, to your diet increases your milk supply and gives you additional energy. To reap beneficial effects you will need to take at least 45 g a day (a heaped tablespoon). Yeast is an acquired taste, but you can mix small amounts of yeast in fruit juice or add it to soups, stews, gravy, scrambled eggs, cereal, or yogurt. This type of yeast is rich in B complex vitamins, protein, and iron. As with dairy products, some women have a sensitivity to yeast. If you have a history of candida (thrush) or food allergy, yeast is probably not for you. Yeast supplements can also make your baby windy.

Fish, especially cold water fish, is a beneficial source of additional protein while you are feeding. This low-fat, protein-packed food is rich in essential fatty acids (EFAs), notably omega-3 fatty acids, which are crucial for your baby's nervous system, brain, and eyes to develop optimally.

If your birthing wounds (in the form of episiotomy, natural tear, or cesarean wound) are slow to heal, and your milk flow just isn't what it should be, your diet may be lacking adequate supplies of zinc. This nutrient is essential for healing, and for the production of breast milk. You are especially likely to be lacking if you are a vegetarian, or exist on a diet of convenience foods, or if you have been using iron supplements throughout your pregnancy, as this mineral hinders the absorption of zinc. Zinc-boosting foods include most seafoods, but especially shellfish; nuts and seeds, especially pumpkin seeds; whole grains; and leafy green vegetables.

You will be passing on large amounts of milk a day to your infant—fluid that must be replaced through your own intake. While you are feeding, try to drink at least eight glasses of water, diluted juice, or herbal tea, each day.

While you are breastfeeding, eat a well-balanced diet and pay special attention to your fluid intake and dietary protein. The following supplements may be used to ensure you are not lacking in any nutrients:

- A multi-mineral supplement containing calcium, magnesium, zinc, and iron, to supply at least 1000 mg of calcium, half as much magnesium, 50 mg of elemental zinc, and 15 mg of iron.

- A multi-vitamin containing vitamins A, the B complex, C, and E, to supply up to 10,000 iu of vitamin A, 50 mg of the main B vitamins, 2000 mg of vitamin C, and 200 to 400 iu of vitamin E.

Watch those Toxins

Besides eating well, try to become aware of the various toxins that you can pass on to your baby through your milk. While you are feeding, do your best not to use pharmacological drugs, and avoid noxious chemicals such as nicotine from cigarettes, alcohol, caffeine from coffee, and recreational drugs such as marijuana. Try to avoid contact with chemicals both in your home and at work. Be especially vigilant to avoid areas that are being sprayed with pesticides or herbicides, and wash all your fruit and vegetables thoroughly before eating them. Even better, switch over to organic fruits and vegetables if you can.

- *Alcohol.* If you drink while you are breastfeeding, your baby receives alcohol through your milk in doses equivalent to your blood alcohol level.

- *Aspirin.* Your baby receives amounts lower than your blood levels, but this drug can still cause stomach upsets in your baby and should not be used in high doses or for prolonged periods of time.

- *Caffeine.* You pass on about one percent of your ingested caffeine through your milk. If you drink coffee, tea, or cola drinks in large amounts, you may find your baby exhibiting irritability and restlessness.

- *Nicotine.* This is excreted through your milk and can cause nausea and vomiting in your baby and decrease your milk supply.

Breast Engorgement and Cracked Nipples

One or two days after the birth, your milk will come in, and you will acquire the most stunning new breast dimensions overnight. Read Chapter 10 on postnatal health problems for some solutions to any discomfort. To avoid cracked nipples make sure that your baby takes the whole areola (brown area) into the mouth when feeding, not just the nipple. The nipple should be well back in baby's mouth to avoid being pressed against his of her hard palate.

Insufficient Milk Supply

After months of disturbed sleep and the constant demands of a small baby, it is not uncommon to find your milk production dropping off, and your baby becoming insatiable. If this happens, check that your good nutritional habits haven't slipped. A daily B complex supplement can help to stimulate your milk production.

Are you getting plenty of rest during the day? Let the housework stay undone. Nourishing your baby is more important than dusting.

Are you drinking enough? The liquid that goes into making breast milk has to come from your fluid intake. If you don't seem to have enough milk, try not to resort to supplementing with formula, as this will further decrease your milk production. The more your baby stimulates your nipples, the more your body will produce milk. Fennel tea and red raspberry tea will help increase and enrich your milk, if drunk several times daily. You could also try adding copious amounts of alfalfa sprouts to your meals, as alfalfa is a notorious milk stimulator.

If nothing seems to help, and you are still intent on breastfeeding, a few appointments with an acupuncturist may solve your problems. Acupuncture is extremely effective for stimulating milk production.

Homeopathic Help To Boost Your Milk Supplies

- *Agnus Castus*. The flow of milk is too short, quickly reducing or stopping shortly after the baby starts feeding. You may often feel and appear weak, with a pale face and anemia.

- *Pulsatilla*. As above, the flow of milk is weak, but this remedy is especially appropriate when milk supply is variable.

- *Causticum*. Weak flow of milk right from the start of feeding. You may appear anxious and tired and suffer from insomnia.

- *Urtica Urens*. This remedy is indicated when there is absolutely no milk being produced. The breasts feel painful with stinging, itching sensations in the breasts.

If you have been breastfeeding successfully until now, and you suspect a particular event has caused your milk production to decrease, maybe one of the following remedies would help you: Aconite is indicated when your milk is suppressed due to a fearful experience, while Chamomilla is the remedy to deal with the results of an excessively fierce, angry outburst. If you have endured a sudden shock or grief, Ignatia is the remedy of choice, while Pulsatilla is indicated if your milk decreases following exposure to the cold or damp.

Traditional Chinese Aids to Milk Production

An old Chinese recipe to stimulate milk production involves boiling 4 or 5 ounces of bean curd (tofu) with a tablespoon of brown sugar and three cups of water. Drink this all at once, once a day for five days. Brown rice, cracked wheat (such as bulghar wheat), and lettuce are all traditionally considered to be milk-producing foods.

Mastitis

Mastitis is the name given to pain and inflammation of the breast caused by infection. Your breast will probably be very tender, red, and hot, and you may well feel tired, run down, and feverish. If you catch your mastitis early enough, you can usually treat yourself using simple home remedies, without having to resort to antibiotics.

You may have developed your infection through a cracked nipple allowing bacteria into your breast. Or perhaps you have been wearing too tight a bra which plugged a milk duct, preventing milk flow and encouraging infection. Whatever the cause of your infection, the important thing now is to rest, sleep whenever possible, *continue breastfeeding from the infected breast*, and start with some of these simple home remedies.

Apply heat to your infected breast as often as possible. One pleasant way is to stand under a hot shower, or soak in a long, hot bath. Wrap a hot-water bottle in a towel and keep it against your sore breast.

When it comes to herbal medicine, the plant supreme for breast infections is pokeroot (Phytolacca). Pokeroot ointment should be massaged over the entire breast, taking great care to avoid getting any on the nipple. This herb may be taken internally in tincture form, but because of its potential toxicity, see a qualified herbalist rather than self-administering.

Mastitis is an infection, and as with all other infections, garlic is a useful herbal remedy. If you wish to use fresh garlic, crush two to three cloves a day and eat them however you can. An easy way to take this pungent herb is to add it crushed to a glass of hot water and lemon juice. You can sweeten the mixture slightly with a little raw honey. If you use a commercial garlic supplement, make sure that you are using a reliable one with a worthwhile potency. Many of the garlic oil preparations for sale contain worthless amounts of garlic floating in a base of soy oil. Reliable supplements include Nature's Way Garlicyn and Kyloic.

Give your immune system the extra boost it needs by following the immune booster program outlined on page 58. If your breast infection continues to worsen over a 48-hour period, despite everything, you must see your doctor, as antibiotics may prove necessary.

Ancient Chinese Cures for Mastitis

Chinese dietary therapy offers some traditional cures for mastitis. These include:

- *Tangerine seeds.* Boil one-half ounce of tangerine seeds in a mixture of half water and half wine. Drink a cup of juice three times a day.

- *Spring onion.* Boil five ounces of white heads of spring onion and two ounces of malt in two cups of water for 20 minutes. Wrap the onion heads and malt in a clean white cloth. While still hot, use them to rub repeatedly along the breast toward the nipple until the breast becomes red and soft. This is an appropriate treatment in the early stages of acute mastitis, before there is any suppuration.

Chapter 12

Menopause— A Change for the Better?

Some time between the ages of approximately 43 and 55 years you will enter that much maligned, often misunderstood stage of your womanhood known as the menopause. The term "menopause" literally means a pause or cessation of the menses—a time when the endless cycle of ovulation and menstruation winds down and then finally stops completely. In those cultures where maturity is revered and respected, women pass through the menopause with a minimum of physical and emotional disruption, simply accepting it as another stage in their natural evolution.

Unfortunately, in Western countries it is not uncommon for women to dread the menopause and to suffer a myriad of mental, emotional, and physical signs of ill health at this time. Some of these side-effects have a sound physiological basis, resulting from seesawing hormonal balances and a drastic reduction in the female hormone estrogen. Others, however, are largely due to the negative conditioning surrounding aging and this society's obsessive preoccupation with youth and beauty.

The media barrages you daily with the message that women (in particular) are only desirable when they are young and "flawless." Female sexuality is displayed and discussed with an intensity and frankness as never before. Periods, contraception, PMS, sexually transmitted diseases all get in-depth coverage and attention. The menopause is treated as the poor sister with relatively little public awareness, a distinct lack of interest from the media, and a large degree of ignorance from society in general.

How you experience your own inevitable menopause is partly up to you. You can choose to accept and move through this change, focusing on the positive aspects such as an end to the inconvenience, mess, pain, and expense of periods; an end to years of worry about unplanned pregnancy and contraceptives; and the beginning of a new era of freedom and lack of child-rearing responsibility. Or you can get caught up in the media con job, and believe the youth cult. The choice is yours.

What Is the Menopause?

To understand the menopause you need to understand the mechanics of your menstrual cycle (explained in Chapter 1). The word menopause is misleading in some ways, implying a condition that occurs for a short time, on exactly the day that the periods stop. The menopause often lasts for two or three years, during which hormonal changes occur which gradually wind down the menstrual cycle. As a female, you are born with tiny ovaries containing your full quotient of eggs—enough to last years of ovulating, with plenty left over. Besides secreting eggs, the ovaries perform the very important function of producing most of your body's female hormone, estrogen. As the total number of eggs left in your ovaries declines, your estrogen production also declines. It is this declining level of estrogen that is largely responsible for the uncomfortable physical symptoms of menopause experienced by some women.

After menopause your body does still produce estrogen, but in much smaller amounts than before. While the ovaries are no longer producing this hormone, your body continues to manufacture small amounts of estrogen from hormones secreted by your adrenal glands. These hormones are changed into estrogen in the fat layers beneath your skin. Interestingly, overweight women produce more estrogen post-menopausally than thin women, and consequently make the transition through menopause with fewer physical symptoms.

What Are the Symptoms of Menopause?

Ideally, the only symptom of menopause is that your periods stop. In reality, many women in Western countries experience a range of physical, mental, and emotional changes besides this. Some women notice changes in their menstrual cycle or pre-menstrual symptoms as early as 35 years of age. This can take the form of worsening PMS, irritability, and breast distention in particular. Prior to periods actually stopping, it is common to notice changes in your menstrual cycle. Your cycle may become longer, with an occasional period missed. Your blood loss may be lighter and perhaps the number of days of bleeding reduced.

In the months (or years) leading up to and after your final period, you may experience any of the following physical symptoms:

- Hot flashes that are characterized by sudden, unbearable, intense heat and drenching sweats

- Dryness and irritation in your vagina

- Dry skin

- Urinary incontinence

- Insomnia

- Psychological symptoms such as anxiety, nervousness, depression, and mood swings.

- Changes in your bone physiology which greatly increase your likelihood of developing osteoporosis, which thins the bones

If you do experience any of these symptoms during the menopause, there are a range of natural and safe solutions besides resorting to estrogen replacement therapy (ERT), a subject we will look at in more detail later.

Hot Flashes

Between 63 and 75 percent of all menopausal women experience hot flashes, ranging in intensity from nothing more than the occasional sensation of heat to frequent drenching sweats that can make life a misery. Flashes are often one of the first symptoms of approaching menopause, sometimes starting well before you notice any changes in menstruation.

So what causes these strange thermostatic breakdowns? No one knows for certain—there are various theories, none of which has been proven conclusively. The most popular theory concerns the hormone LH (luteinizing hormone) which served you for years triggering the release of the egg from your ovary each month. During and after your menopause LH levels rise, but they often surge, and it is this surge that is thought to trigger body changes with the end result a hot flash.

If you are experiencing these flashes, there are some simple, common sense things you can do to make them easier to deal with. For example, try to dress in layers each day (choosing especially natural fibers which allow your body to "breathe"), so that you can take off as many layers as necessary when you experience a flash. When you get a flash, breathe deeply, relax, and try not to panic. Although they may feel terrible, they are in no way dangerous or harmful. Try to avoid warming substances such as strong coffee, alcohol, and spicy dishes such as curry, and tobacco.

Nutritional Therapy

When it comes to hot flashes, two nutritional supplements stand out—vitamin E and selenium. Bioflavinoids are also reputed to have beneficial effects on this problem.

Vitamin E, taken in doses of between 400 and 1200 iu a day, has been shown in trials (and endorsed by millions of menopausal women) to be effective in stopping hot flashes. Its effects are usually noticed within a month to six weeks of starting supplementation. Start supplementing with small amounts, say 400 iu a day, of mixed tocopherol vitamin E. This is best taken after a meal, and well after any iron supplements you may be taking, as iron destroys this vitamin. Gradually increase your dosage, over a period of a week, to 800 iu a day. If this fails to help, keep increasing the dose to up to 1200 iu a day. If you don't get immediate results, remain on this high dose for three or four weeks before giving up on the treatment. Vitamin E can be toxic in very high doses, so do not be tempted to keep increasing the dose to ever greater heights. If you are diabetic, have high blood pressure, or are taking medication, consult your doctor before you start using this supplement in high doses.

The trace element selenium is missing from many soils. It can be toxic, although small doses of up to 100 mcg a day can be taken safely, in conjunction with vitamin E. It is a potent anti-oxidant, protecting the cell walls in your body and preventing premature aging and cell abnormalities such as cancer.

Bioflavinoids are found in your diet, most commonly in citrus fruits. This substance greatly enhances the absorption and utilization of vitamin C, as well as strengthening the walls of your blood capillaries. Bioflavinoids can help you control your hot flashes. Doses anywhere from 500 mg to 2000 mg of bioflavinoids can be taken daily, along with vitamin C (500 mg to 2000 mg a day).

A balanced high potency B complex is another useful part of your nutritional management of this problem. These vitamins are essential for the healthy functioning of your nervous system, and will increase your ability to withstand stress (including the stress of your menopausal symptoms).

Herbal Help

A number of female hormonal regulator herbs are used to help reduce the severity and frequency of hot flashes. These include black cohosh, false unicorn root, damiana, motherwort, passion flower, squaw vine, and chastetree. The Chinese herb ginseng is effective because of its natural stimulation of estrogen production. Another Chinese herb, dong quai, is also traditionally used for menopausal hormonal imbalances. Dong quai, taken as a dried herb or tincture, helps lower blood pressure, prevent vaginal dryness, ensure regular bowel movements, and boost your energy. It is not suitable for every woman. Some find it produces symptoms like PMS, with nervousness and anxiety. See a qualified medical herbalist if you wish to use herbs to deal with the effects of your shifting hormones.

Homeopathic Treament of Hot Flashes

- *Belladonna*. Indicated for intense hot flashes with reddening and burning of the face, accompanied by restlessness and irritability. There may also be palpitations, and all symptoms are made worse by any kind of movement, touch, or jarring.

- *Lachesis.* A very important remedy for hot flashes that are accompanied by sweating and severe headaches centered on the top of the scalp. The flashes and headaches are worse in the morning and worse for sleep. Lachesis patients cannot stand any kind of pressure on their bodies, such as a tight waist band.

- *Pulsatilla.* For the very emotional woman who is prone to fits of crying and bothered by mild hot flashes that come and go quickly. Symptoms are made worse by any kind of heat.

Vaginal Dryness

As your estrogen levels drop, your vagina gradually becomes shorter and less elastic. The blood supply to the vagina also decreases, and the mucous membranes lining it become more fragile and prone to infection. The vaginal lubrication also decreases noticeably and in some women this leads to a permanent sensation of dryness, soreness, and a lack of interest in sexual intercourse. Your doctor will probably offer you estrogen ointment to insert into the vagina, and while it is true that this therapy certainly makes a difference to your vagina, it is not without its drawbacks. Substantial amounts of estrogen are absorbed through the vaginal lining into the bloodstream, and as you will see later, supplementing with synthetic estrogen can have some hazardous side-effects.

One of the most effective ways of preventing this problem is to enjoy an active sex life. Regular intercourse and orgasms have been proven to keep your vaginal membranes thicker and stronger. If you don't have a partner, don't despair—the same research shows that masturbation to orgasm has the same beneficial effects on your vagina. For more information on preventing and dealing with vaginal infections, see the section on thrush in the A-Z. All the advice given there is relevant for coping with infections during the menopausal years, too.

If you suffer from vaginal dryness, there are some common sense practical steps to take in conjunction with the various nutritional and herbal solutions outlined later.

- Avoid using soap, bubble baths, douches, and personal hygiene products. They all tend to dry the vaginal area and can cause irritation.

- Avoid tight-fitting underwear and wear only cotton underpants. If you wear pantyhose, buy those with a cotton panty or no panty! Ventilation will help prevent thrush outbreaks. Whenever you can, around home, go without any underwear at all.

- Use a personal lubricant during sexual intercourse, and spend adequate time in foreplay. The same vitamin E that helps you deal with hot flashes is useful in coping with a dry vagina. The oil-filled capsules can be pierced and applied locally to the outside and inside of the vagina.

Vitamin E should also be taken orally at the same time, in doses of up to 800 iu a day.

- Some women swear by regular douching with natural *Lactobacillus* yogurt. The same effect can be obtained, but with decidedly less mess, by inserting lactobacillus capsules high into your vagina at night.

Homeopathic Remedies for Vaginal Thinning and Dryness

- *Nat Mur.* For dryness of the internal membranes causing severe pain in the vagina, often accompanied by depression and tearfulness.

- *Bryonia.* For vaginal dryness accompanied by severe constipation and often a dry cough or sore throat.

- *Staphisagria.* For dry, thin vaginal membranes damaged through intercourse that results in severe pain and feelings of anger and resentment.

Insomnia

As you age, you need fewer hours of sleep, but you still do need *some* sleep, and of good quality. If you are experiencing restlessness and insomnia at night, and you're in your late forties or your fifties, it may well be due to hormonal imbalance. Try to avoid the temptation of sleeping tablets. They are strongly habit forming and in a short time reduce your natural capacity to experience sound sleep. You may simply need to make some changes to your routine, or may need a little nutritional or herbal help.

Before you go to bed, try to get into the right frame of mind for falling asleep. This means going to bed in a relaxed state, not stewing over the dramas of the day. Try a hot bath, perhaps with candles and some soothing music. An herbal bath can provide even more relaxation because of the therapeutic effects of the herbs. Taking herbal baths can be as simple as throwing in a couple of teaspoons of dried herbs, although this type of bath usually needs to be followed by a shower to wash off all the clinging herbs. The easier option is to take five minutes to make a bath bag. Cut a 12-inch square of cheesecloth or muslin. Fill it with herbs of your choice (see the list below), then gather all the corners together and tie with a string. You can either tie the bag to the tap in the flow of water, or simply allow it to bob around the bathtub with you. If your bag contains dried herbs, it can be used for two or three baths before the herbs need changing. Fresh herbs must be thrown away after each soak.

Another way of making a herbal bath is to add half a pint of your favorite herbal tea to your bath water. Use a china or pottery teapot. Pour the boiling water onto three or four teaspoons of fresh, or one or two teaspoons of dried, herbs. Let it infuse for half an hour, and then strain before adding to the bath water. You can make double the quantity and keep half in a glass screw-top jar for up to one week in the fridge. Your choice of herbs is vast, but these suggestions may be useful.

- A beautifully scented and relaxing combination includes lavender flowers, lemon balm, elder flowers, and rosemary leaves. Lavender is especially useful if you have a headache.

- A chamomile, valerian, or hops bath will leave you feeling truly unwound.

Chamomile or relaxing teas can be taken as your nightcap, and are useful to drink through the evening in place of stimulating caffeine drinks such as coffee, tea, and hot chocolate. Beware the trap of drinking yourself to sleep with alcohol. You may fall asleep more easily, but chances are you won't sleep through the night. Herbal teas are more reliable and lasting relaxants.

If you are feeling tired during the day because of poor night sleep, try to resist the urge to nap. Even as little as half an hour during the day can take the edge off your tiredness at night. Instead, force yourself outside for fresh air and exercise, perhaps a brisk walk along a beach, in a park, or wherever else you find enjoyable. Half an hour to an hour of aerobic exercise each day will usually see your nocturnal habits improve immensely.

If you eat dinner at 6 p.m. and then don't eat again through the evening (maybe you're also battling middle-age spread), by the time you get to bed you may well be suffering the ill effects of low blood sugar. When this happens, you feel tense and jittery and unable to relax enough to sleep. Ensure against this by having a mid-evening snack of slow-burning complex carbohydrates such as a small bowl of oatmeal, or a slice of whole grain bread, or a little rice pudding or pasta.

The amino acid tryptophan used to be one of the most frequently prescribed solutions to insomnia. In the last couple of years, however, supplements containing tryptophan have been removed from the market, pending further scientific trials. There has been some evidence to suggest it can cause a serious blood disease when taken in high doses. You can still boost your tryptophan levels naturally by including rich sources such as milk, yogurt, bananas, dates, tuna, and peanut butter in your daily diet. This amino acid is used by the brain to create a sleep-inducing chemical called serotonin.

The B complex vitamins and the minerals calcium and magnesium have recognized sleep-inducing properties. Taking a B complex tablet and a balanced calcium and magnesium combination just before bed with a glass of warm milk (if you don't have a lactose intolerance!) can usually overcome even the most stubborn cases of insomnia.

Mood Swings and Depression

In menopause you may also notice a change in your emotional disposition. Even if you have previously prided yourself on your calm and collected temperment, you may suddenly find yourself acting like a stranger. Seesawing emotions, inexplicable anxiety, depression, and almost phobic fears can result from your rapidly changing hormonal balance. You may experience emotional symptoms similar to PMS or postnatal depression—two other problems related to hormonal readjustments.

Some women cruise through menopause with their normal sweet disposition, while others turn into nervous wrecks. Although individual biochemistry partly determines which category you fall into, some aspects are within your control. If you smoke, drink alcohol regularly, consume large amounts of coffee, live on junk food, or indulge a sweet tooth constantly, your chances are far greater of falling into the nervous wreck category.

Depression around your menopausal years is often also related to the strange disrespect accorded to middle-aged women. Youth and beauty are held up as barometers of value and self-esteem. When the wrinkles start to appear and your midriff expands you suddenly realize you no longer live up to the unrealistic image of perpetual perfection. Even if you have previously managed to escape acknowledging the march of time, when you enter the menopause you are suddenly faced with an irrefutable, concrete sign of aging.

You may also, for the first time in your life, have absolutely no excuses for not getting on with the things that you have talked about for years, but never quite managed to do; for example, furthering your education, getting a better job, leaving an unhappy marriage. Your children are probably grown and independent and for the first time in perhaps 20 or 30 years you have time to sit back and take stock of your life. Being faced with choices, new options, and the chance to express your independence and freedom can be daunting and unsettling.

Sexual difficulties or a feeling of insecurity and uncertainty regarding your own sexuality are also common around the menopause. You may suddenly feel much less sexually attractive, and less interested in sex. Physical difficulties such as a dry vagina and repeated vaginal and urinary tract infections are also a definite turnoff, perhaps making sex unpleasant and painful for you. With all of this combined, it's hardly surprising if you experience some emotional upheavals along with your physical ones.

So how do you deal with it? Start by defining your own parameters for valuing yourself. Forget the media and the general ignorance and shortsightedness regarding the menopause that pervades society. Learn to love yourself and value yourself for all the positive qualities you possess. Look within for your positive reinforcement and worry less about others' attitudes or lack of sensitivity. Focusing on your new-found freedom, mid-life prosperity, and opportunity to develop friendships and personal relationships with other women and men will override the usual negative publicity surrounding your changes. Whatever happens, if you can't manage your anxiety or mood swings, don't be afraid to turn to others for help. Talk to other women who may be experiencing the same difficulties, or older friends who have weathered the storm already. Talk to your partner, sharing books about the menopause and encouraging greater understanding and emotional support. Turn to professionals for advice, perhaps an understanding counselor or a health care professional that you know and trust.

If at all possible, try to resist the easy solution of using tranquilizers and anti-depressants. If you visit your doctor specifically to talk about your emotional problems, he or she will most probably try to prescribe these or ERT. Think very carefully before you accept either. Tranquilizers are the most widely used prescription drug ever made. They are also extremely addictive and cause a range of unpleasant side-effects including fatigue, drowsiness, reduced sex drive, nausea, irritability, and (yes!) depression. Tranquilizers and anti-depressants also mask your symptoms, providing you with a useful way of avoiding addressing the problems and underlying difficulties in your life. Before resorting to these powerful drugs, explore every avenue of non-drug therapy available to you.

Self-Help and Natural Therapies

One of the most useful places to start your assault on your depression and anxiety is with an examination of your diet. Is it a nutrient-rich feast of whole foods, or a diet of worthless junk food, refined carbohydrates, and sugar? If it is the latter, don't be too surprised by your erratic moods.

What you put in your mouth can really make a tremendous difference to your emotional balance. Besides lacking sufficient nutrients, junk food diets also contain large amounts of simple carbohydrates and sugar that play havoc with your blood sugar levels. Whenever you eat a cake, cookie, candy bar, sweet, piece of white bread, or other refined carbohydrate, your blood sugar performs somersaults. The food is quickly broken down in your body, releasing a large flood of sugar into your bloodstream. This immediately sends panic signals to your pancreas, which in turn quickly pumps out large amounts of the hormone insulin. This hormone is responsible for taking the excess sugar out of your bloodstream and into your cells. The trouble is, the sudden burst of blood sugar often triggers an overcompensation from your pancreas, which pumps out too much insulin too quickly. The sugar in your blood is rapidly shunted into your cells, often with the end result of a dramatic lowering of your blood sugar. When this happens you experience a range of unpleasant symptoms, including exhaustion, palpitations, sweating, anxiety, irritability, depression, headaches, and tremors. If you subsist on a junk diet, this stressful scenario can be repeated many times a day with very real detrimental effects on your nervous system and mood.

Avoid this situation by cutting out all refined carbohydrates, including white bread, white rice, white pasta, cookies, candies, sugar in any form, sugar-laden breakfast cereals, etc. In their place develop a taste for the more satisfying, unrefined carbohydrates supplied by whole grain bread, brown rice, whole wheat pasta, fresh fruits, and starchy vegetables such as potato, pumpkin, and yams. This type of carbohydrate is broken down slowly, supplying you with a gradually released and sustained supply of sugar (energy). Instead of peaking and troughing, your blood sugar gently rises and maintains the increased levels for a long period of time before gently falling again in time for your next meal. Simply making this one change can often produce immediate, dramatic improvement in your energy, sense of well-being, and mood.

If you have always been a three-meals-a-day person, try changing your eating routine to six mini-meals instead. Eat breakfast, lunch, and dinner, with a high-quality nutritional snack in between. There is no need to increase your overall intake of food, just redistribute it and cut down on the amount consumed at each sitting. "Grazing," as this type of eating has become known, has been shown to be beneficial for human physiology, and ensures a sustained and adequate amount of sugar in your blood at all times. This in turn results in a feeling of increased energy, clearer mental functioning, and a balance in your emotional well-being.

Make your snacks count nutritionally, choosing from a wide range of proteins, complex carbohydrates, and high-fiber foods such as fruits and vegetables. Your mini-meals need be no more complex than eating a handful of mixed nuts and seeds, or a pear, or a piece of whole grain bread with a little low-fat cheese or peanut butter. Low-fat yogurts, fresh fruit, cold chicken, or homemade vegetable soup provide other easy options.

If you are suffering from depression or emotional seesaws it may be that you need more of certain nutrients. Although you obtain sufficient nutrients from your daily food intake to keep you alive, you don't always obtain the larger amounts of certain nutrients needed when you are experiencing emotional and physical stress. The hormonal and emotional ups and downs of menopause are very real stressors, and at this time your requirements for the "nervous system" nutrients increase dramatically. In particular you need more of the B complex vitamins, vitamin C, and the minerals calcium and magnesium, which are also needed to stave off the progression of osteoporosis after menopause.

The following nutritional supplements may help you reduce or eliminate anxiety and depression during menopause. Take all supplements with food, in split doses (that is, twice a day rather than in one dose).

- *High potency B complex* supplying 50 mg of most of the B vitamins. Some B complex supplements also contain 500 mg of vitamin C, another vitamin indicated for this problem.

- *Vitamin C* sodium ascorbate (if you don't have high blood pressure), or ascorbic acid (if you don't have problems with excessive stomach acidity or gastric ulcers). Vitamin C tolerance varies: while some people get diarrhea after only 1000 mg of C, others can take 5000 mg without any problems. You need about 1000 mg of C a day, taken in split doses of 500 mg twice daily. High doses of vitamin C, while in no way harmful, have been shown to increase the leaching of calcium from your bones. If you want to take higher doses, use the calcium ascorbate form (this is not necessary if you are also taking a multi-mineral formula).

- *Multi-mineral formula* containing a balanced ratio of calcium and magnesium (two parts calcium to one part magnesium). Use formulas that supply chelated or orotate minerals, which are readily utilized by your body. This should be taken twice daily, to supply at least 1000 mg of calcium and 500 mg of magnesium.

Herbal Help

Herbal help for the nervous system falls into three main groups:

- Herbs to strengthen the nervous system (nervine tonics)
- Herbs to relax and ease nervous tension (nervine relaxants)
- Herbs to stimulate the nervous system (nervine stimulants).

In cases of anxiety, depression, and tension it is appropriate to use both the tonics and relaxants. One of the best herbs for nourishing and strengthening the nervous system is the humble oat, which can be taken as an herbal remedy or as a food. It is rich in calcium and silica, and is specifically indicated if there is nervous debility and exhaustion along with depression.

The relaxant herbs are appropriate to use in cases of ongoing stress, tension, and an inability to relax. As well as those herbs already discussed under the section on insomnia, other nervines include black cohosh, hyssop, lady's slipper, lime blossom, rosemary, and skullcap. These herbs are most effective when taken in appropriate combinations, and for this reason consulting an herbalist is preferable to self-administering. This doesn't stop you from using calming herbal teas such as lemon balm and chamomile, and using relaxing herbs in your bathwater.

Exercise and Meditation

Eating properly is only half the picture when it comes to dealing with any health problems, and depression and anxiety are no exception. Regular aerobic exercise has been proven to stimulate the production of mood-elevating chemicals in the brain (endorphins), and significantly reduce nervousness, anxiety, depression, and mood swings. This effect seems to be ongoing, meaning that it doesn't just occur for the short period of time during which you are actually exercising.

Aerobic exercise need not mean putting on a leotard and joining the local gym (although by all means do so, if it appeals). Something as simple as a brisk walk for 40 minutes, three times a week, is enough to reap beneficial rewards. Using an exercycle or jumping on a mini trampoline, gentle jogging, or swimming are other useful alternatives.

Try to make the time to practice some form of relaxation or meditation regularly. Your relaxation may be walking in the fresh air, gardening, having a hot bath, or listening to music. Whatever calms you, make the time to do it. Get into the habit of spending five minutes going through the progressive relaxation exercise outlined in Chapter 4 before you turn out the lights at night. It will help you sleep more soundly and in turn your days will also be less tense.

Menopause and Your Diet—
Meeting Your Special Needs

While the basic principles of healthy eating apply as much during menopause as at any other time of your life, several specific nutrients will help you pass this landmark with minimal disruption to your body and mind. Some of these, such as B complex vitamins and vitamins E and C, have already been discussed. Other important menopausal nutrients include bioflavinoids, essential fatty acids, and magnesium and calcium.

Susan Lark in her *Menopause Self-Help Book* sings the praises of bioflavinoids, stating that along with vitamin E, they should be called the "menopause vitamin." She points out that bioflavinoids have chemical activity similar to estrogen, and can be used as an estrogen substitute, without the harmful side-effects characteristic of ERT. As well as providing relief from hot flashes, anxiety, irritability, and mood swings, bioflavinoids can also effectively reduce blood loss in women with excessively heavy periods (as is so common during the time leading up to menopause). Easy bruising and bleeding gums are two other signs that you need more of this nutrient. Bioflavinoids are found specifically in the white pith of citrus fruits, and also in buckwheat.

Calcium and magnesium are two of the minerals most important for building and maintaining a healthy skeleton. When your estrogen production diminishes, calcium is leached from your bones at a faster rate than before. If you have survived many years on a calcium-deficient diet, your bones will be less dense than they could be, and consequently you will be more likely to suffer the ravages of osteoporosis after menopause. There has been much contention over whether taking calcium and magnesium supplements during and after the menopause makes any difference to your likelihood of developing this bone-thinning disease. Most of the evidence now indicates that indeed it's never too late to start looking after your bones. Read the section on osteoporosis in the A-Z for a more detailed look at the role of calcium in preventing this disease.

Your calcium requirements during menopause rocket to around 1200 to 1500 mg a day—an amount that's difficult to supply through dietary sources alone. Of course you should eat plenty of the high-calcium foods such as green leafy vegetables, bony fish, seeds, nuts, and some dairy products, but you also need to be using a balanced calcium supplement daily. The most effective supplements are those containing a range of synergistic minerals (that is, minerals that work together to enhance each other's absorption and utilization) such as calcium, magnesium, silica, phosphorus, and vitamin D. Use orotate, chelate, or citrate forms of calcium to ensure adequate absorption, and take your supplements on an empty stomach, along with a glass of fruit juice.

As well as benefiting your skeleton, adequate calcium supplies also help guard against high blood pressure and excessive blood fats (both of which contribute to heart disease). The magnesium you get from your mineral supplement will also help combat some other menopausal problems you may experience. For example, magnesium helps to regulate your sugar metabolism and reduce blood sugar swings, thus reducing the fatigue that many menopausal women complain of. Through its effects on your brain chemistry, this mineral also elevates your mood and prevents mood swings and depression.

If you feel as if you're drying up with brittle hair, parchment skin, and a dry vagina, you need to pay attention to your essential fatty acid (EFA) intake. These fats can't be manufactured by your body and so must be supplied through your daily intake of food. All your body's cells use essential fatty acids to build strong cell walls. Your adrenal glands, so important for supplying that little bit of estrogen after your menopause, also need these fats.

Essential fatty acids in the form of evening primrose oil have received widespread and favorable publicity in relation to their beneficial effects in women with PMS. It is these same essential fatty acids (linoleic and linolenic acid) that ease menopausal dryness, and at the same time decrease your risk of heart disease by decreasing the stickiness of your blood and regulating your blood pressure.

So where do you get these EFAs from? Besides investing in a bottle of evening primrose oil from your local health food shop, you can ensure a daily intake by using cold-pressed vegetable oils, such as sesame seed oil, sunflower seed oil, corn oil, wheat germ oil, but especially flax seed oil (not to be found on your average supermarket shelf!), and consuming several servings of oily fish such as salmon, tuna, and mackerel each week. Make sure that you take your oil in its natural, unheated state, as cooking destroys the essential fatty acids. Use the oil to make salad dressings, or add a teaspoon or so to your food for flavoring after it is cooked. To combat menopausal problems you may need up to two tablespoons a day. If this seems like a horrendous amount of oil, you may find it easier to supply some of your requirements with four capsules of evening primrose oil each day. If you increase your dietary intake of fats, you must also increase your intake of vitamin E. Many EPO (Evening Primrose Oil) supplements also contain vitamin E.

Diet Is Just Half the Story . . .

So far, most of the focus on dealing with menopausal problems has been on eating the right food and taking the right nutritional or herbal supplements. Certainly this approach to staying healthy is important, but it is only half of the equation. As well as putting the right fuel in your body, you also need to make your body work for its keep. That entails regular (but not necessarily exhausting) exercise. On its own, exercise can help prevent (or improve) many of the common menopausal problems such as hot flashes, mood swings, urinary tract and vaginal infections, insomnia, osteoporosis, and your increased risk of heart disease.

Many of your "down below" problems result from your falling levels of estrogen. However, these problems are worsened through lack of physical activity and the resultant poor muscle tone and lack of blood circulation in your lower abdomen. The simple solution is two or three sessions of vigorous exercise each week. If you enjoy swimming, grab your towel. Hop on your bike if that's what you prefer; put on your running shoes, or simply pound the pavement at a brisk walk.

One of the most effective exercises for improving blood circulation and tone in your pelvic area is lovemaking. When it comes to the health of your vagina during menopause, the old adage "use it or lose it" certainly seems to apply. Women who make love or masturbate regularly are much less troubled by dry, irritated vagina and infections.

The other specific exercises for your pelvic organs are pelvic floor or kegel exercises. These exercises are simple to do and are described in detail in Chapter 3. Make them a part of your daily routine. They can be done anywhere and at any time—washing the dishes, sitting at your desk, or in front of the television.

When you exercise aerobically, your blood pumps vigorously around your body, nourishing and oxygenating all your muscles, internal organs, and your brain. Calming (almost sedative) hormones called endorphins are released by your brain in response to your activity. These partly explain the feeling of relaxation and well-being after a 30- or 40-minute walk or jog. Endorphins and increased blood supply to your brain greatly reduce the likelihood of you suffering the tortures of mood swings, depression, and insomnia.

It has been proven that the skeleton benefits from exercising. If you seriously want a strong, healthy skeleton as you grow old, you need to do more than pop an occasional calcium tablet. Adequate calcium intake is important to prevent osteoporosis, but equally important is the regular exercise your body needs to fix the calcium into your bones. You lose the most calcium from your bones during times of inactivity—this includes the time when you are sleeping. People who are immobilized because of illness lose greatly increased amounts of calcium in their urine.

The most effective exercise for strengthening your bones is weight-bearing exercise—that is, exercise in which your body exercises against some kind of resistance. For the bones of your lower body this could be walking, running, dancing, or golfing; and for your upper body, tennis, racquetball, or weight-lifting (even using two large cans of dog food as weights can provide enough resistance to strengthen your arm bones).

Before you reach the menopause the odds of you dying of a heart attack are relatively slim compared with your male partner of a similar age (providing you don't smoke or use the contraceptive pill, and aren't dramatically overweight). This male/female difference diminishes somewhat after the menopause, and exercise becomes an increasingly important part of maintaining your cardiovascular health. Regular aerobic exercise encourages your heart and lungs to perform more efficiently. Exercise also dilates and expands the tiny blood vessels in your body, which in turn increases the flow of oxygen and nutrients to your muscles and organs.

You've heard plenty about the dangers of excessive blood fat levels, and exercising is one of the most efficient ways of lowering these cholesterol levels (along with a sensible diet). The brisk walking or jogging you perform to strengthen your bones will provide all these benefits for your cardiovascular system. The ideal is about 45 minutes of brisk walking, three times weekly. See your doctor before embarking on any new fitness program, especially if you have been unfit for a long time.

Estrogen or Hormone Replacement Therapy (ERT or HRT)

Today's menopausal women are among the first generations of women who have had a choice when it comes to menopause. They can choose to pass through the menopause without the assistance of pharmacological intervention, dealing in whatever way they can with any unpleasant symptoms that may occur along the way. Or they can choose to intervene in nature's plan for their hormones, by using synthetic estrogen replacements.

HRT is an emotional and sensitive topic, with firm camps on both sides of the argument for and against its use. For the pharmaceutical companies that manufacture it, and the doctors who prescribe it, it is potentially a huge and never-ending well of revenue. Once you begin taking HRT you must undertake regular visits to your doctor for tests, observation, and possible alteration of your estrogen dose.

Despite much research with clear conclusions, there is still widespread confusion and misinformation regarding exactly which menopausal problems HRT is an effective solution for. The advertising literature claims it reduces your chances of osteoporosis, heart disease, mood swings and anxiety, and vaginal and bladder problems, including dryness and increased tendency to infections. There are even implications that HRT will serve as some kind of panacea against aging; rather like a modern-day "youth pill."

In 1971 the Department of Health, Education, and Welfare published a report that was the result of a huge conference on the subject. It states that "Only hot flashes and genital atrophy [drying and thinning of the vagina] are unique clinical features of the menopause and these are responsive to low dose estrogen therapy." In other words there is no proof that HRT will do anything for your mood swings, anxiety, weight gain, skin wrinkling, or general aging (despite what the advertising literature may tell you).

A British study carried out over a six-month period supports this finding. Half of the women were given HRT while the other half received a dummy sugar pill, or placebo. Each woman was carefully monitored for any changes in her menopausal symptoms including hot flashes, depression, insomnia, dizziness, headaches, joint pain, and nervousness. By the end of the study it was clear that there was no difference in the improvement of symptoms of the two groups. Both groups improved equally, while the estrogen replacement group showed a slightly greater improvement in the incidence and severity of hot flashes.

One of the strongest selling points for long-term HRT use is its potential to prevent bone fractures. There is no doubt that HRT slows bone loss after menopause—although this does not necessarily mean that every post-menopausal woman should be using HRT for bone protection (as the pharmaceutical companies are increasingly coming to recommend). HRT slows bone loss only during use; as soon as HRT therapy is discontinued, bone loss accelerates again. Accordingly, long-term use of HRT, from five years upwards, is the type advocated to prevent osteoporosis. With long-term use comes a potential escalation in serious side-effects (many of which may still be largely unknown).

When deciding whether to use HRT for osteoporosis prevention, it is important to evaluate each individual woman's potential risk. Women falling in high-risk categories (as discussed in the section on osteoporosis on pages 243–247) may be better candidates for HRT use than those women with a low likelihood of bone fractures. Over her lifetime, a women in the low-risk category has a 4 percent risk of hip fracture and a 14 percent of vertebral fracture. Since long-term HRT use is estimated to reduce the risk of fracture by 50 percent, for women in the low-risk group its use translates to a 2 percent reduction in hip fractures and a 7 percent reduction in vertebral fractures. One must question whether this fractional reduction in an already low risk can be reconciled with the potentially negative consequences of long-term HRT use. Keep in mind, too, that by far the most sensible way of dealing with osteoporosis is to apply the myriad of lifestyle changes (discussed on pages 243–247) that are known to reduce the incidence of bone-thinning disease. Sensible dietary practices and regular weight-bearing exercise in the pre-menopausal and post-menopausal years will greatly reduce the dangers of osteoporosis.

HRT *does* take away your hot flashes, but once you stop taking it, the flashes will return, sometimes with a fiercer intensity than before. Using HRT simply delays the occurrence of your hot flashes, rather than curing them.

Another proven area of effectiveness is the effect of HRT on the health of your vagina and bladder. Taking estrogen rapidly returns your genitals to their pre-menopausal condition, complete with thicker cell linings, suppleness, and plentiful lubrication. Estrogen for this purpose can be taken orally, or applied to the area as a topical ointment. It used to be thought that the creams were without danger, but it is now clear that estrogen is absorbed from the ointment, through the lining of the vagina and into the bloodstream. Consequently, the risks inherent in using oral estrogen should be considered to apply to the use of estrogen creams also.

Along with osteoporosis prevention, cardiovascular protection is the other main reason for long-term use of HRT. Before menopause, women have much lower rates of heart disease than men, but this advantage begins to diminish after menopause, as declining estrogen levels result in an increase in blood cholesterol and potentially harmful LDL fats. The majority of the research showing the dramatic protective effects of estrogen has been based on the use of ERT with no additional progesterone. It is possible that the addition of progesterone decreases the extent of the protection that estrogen provides, since progesterone decreases "good" HDL cholesterol and increases "bad" LDL fats, and in so doing may rule out any potential benefit from estrogen.

Once again, all the HRT hype makes it easy to forget that we are not all just sitting targets waiting to picked off by heart disease. Rather than advocate an across-the-board use of HRT for cardiovascular protection, individual risk factors should be taken into consideration. Remember, too, that much can be done through lifestyle and diet changes to protect against heart disease. Something as simple as a daily dose of 100 iu of vitamin E has been shown to reduce heart disease among women by a dramatic 46 percent.

So now that you know what HRT can do for you, it's time to consider the down side to the equation. The potential short-term and long-term side effects associated with HRT are well documented, although some of these are more annoying than life threatening. Breast tenderness and a return of PMS are common problems, as is nausea, which usually passes after a few weeks. Many women complain of weight gain and fluid retention. Other common problems include headaches, cramps, heavy periods, bleeding, and feelings of aggression, anxiety, and irritability.

Then there are the potentially more serious risks associated with HRT use. Although study continues into the safety of long-term use, current research is contradictory, and a great deal of contention remains.

Women using estrogen after the menopause have a risk of developing problems with gallstones two and a half times higher than the risk for other women.

Does HRT contribute to the development of cancer? In many instances, the research continues to be inconclusive and confusing. It is now clear that using estrogen replacement therapy (not balanced with additional progesterone) is contraindicated in women who still have a uterus, due to the dramatic increase in endometrial cancer (cancer of the lining of the uterus). The addition of progesterone, however, seems to lower endometrial cancer rates below the rates of women who do not use HRT. For breast cancer the results are far less clear, with some studies showing no correlation between HRT use and breast cancer, and others showing just the contrary. Two major studies carried out in Sweden and England (using a combined total of 27,500 women as the research group) have shown that the risk of breast cancer is 1.8 times greater after using HRT for six years. It is certain that a history of fibrocyctic breast disease or breast cancer is a contraindication for the use of HRT.

There are some clear contraindications for the use of HRT. Of these, cancer of the breast or endometrium or severe liver disease are the only absolute contraindications. The risks for other factors are based more on circumstantial evidence, rather than absolute certainty, and are assessed on an individual basis. Contraindications include:

- Blood-clotting disorders now or in the past

- Stroke or history of any cardiovascular disease including high blood pressure

- Impaired liver function

- Diabetes
- Fibrocystic breast disease
- High blood cholesterol levels
- Cancer of the breast, skin, or reproductive organs
- Fibroids
- Migranes
- Gallstones.

If you decide to go ahead and use HRT, there are certain measures you can take to minimize the dangers to yourself. First and foremost, adopt a sensible attitude to the use of this drug. Don't believe the advertising material promoting HRT as a long-term panacea and an elixir for eternal youth. The truth is that we still don't know what the risks of long-term HRT use are. Most of our knowledge is based on studies of short-term use (from six months to five years), and even then much of the research is unclear.

If you are using ERT (or any other pharmacological drug), you can safeguard yourself by taking some of the responsibility for your health. You are just one of hundreds of patients seen by your doctor. Take the initiative by insisting on a thorough checkup and reappraisal of the need for using HRT, every six months. Why continue to use a synthetic steroid drug any longer than necessary? Also, be alert for any changes in your body. In particular pay attention to any vaginal bleeding or thickening or lumpiness of the breasts.

Pay special attention to your diet and acknowledge your increased nutritional requirements while using ERT. Read Chapter 6 on the nutritional consequences of using the pill, and embark on the nutritional regime outlined.

I am a strong believer in using pharmaceutical drugs only as a last resort, and I feel no differently on the subject of HRT. Be aware that complementary therapies have much to offer women experiencing difficulties going through the natural transitional period of the menopause. Remember, too, that generations of women have passed through the menopause without the assistance of HRT and lived to tell the tale!

Are There Any Natural Alternatives to HRT?

Estrogen replacement therapy is an artificial attempt at returning your hormonal balance to its pre-menopausal state and in so doing alleviate all your bothersome symptoms associated with menopause. Stop for a minute and consider that this therapy is totally contrary to the natural design of nature that has ruled the ebb and flow of female cycles since the beginning of time. Women were not designed to go on menstruating and bearing children throughout their lives, and the menopause is the natural demarcation of release from reproductive life.

Consider, too, that many women pass through the menopause with no physical or emotional problems. These are the women who reach the menopausal years in a high state of wellness, both physically and emotionally. They have no need for HRT because they have no problematic symptoms associated with the cessation of their periods. Thus, nature's alternative to HRT is an emphasis on total wellness to attain the highest possible level of health and well-being and thus pass through this turning point without incidence.

And how does one achieve this wellness? Through applying the basic principles espoused in this and many other natural health books—the principles of sound nutrition, peace of mind, and regular exercise. Your mental attitude to menopause will also influence your experience of this process. Viewing menopause as an end or a loss of youth, reproductive ability, and validation of self is almost guaranteed to see you winding up with a plethora of unpleasant physical and emotional symptoms at this time. In more primitive (and in many ways more enlightened) cultures, women pass through the menopause without incident, partly because of their different attitude to aging. In cultures where older women are revered and appreciated for their wisdom and life experience, menopause is almost inconsequential.

Chapter 13

Complementary Therapies

The last 10 years have seen a huge upsurge in the number and variety of complementary therapies available in Western countries. There has been an associated change in the attitude of many (both lay people and those involved in the conventional medical scene), with a broadening of minds and a willingness to explore these somewhat less conventional methods of healing. Some complementary therapies have even been embraced by the established system, with acupuncture and osteopathy, for instance, receiving coverage by some private medical insurance companies. More and more doctors are willing to refer their patients to trained and qualified acupuncturists, osteopaths, chiropractors, and homeopaths for treatment.

Within the field of complementary medicine not all therapies stand equally acknowledged and accepted by society. Some complementary therapies have long histories of healing, and are generally more widely accepted than others. These include:

- Acupuncture
- Medical herbalism
- Homeopathy
- Naturopathy
- Osteopathy
- Chiropractic.

The twentieth century has seen the emergence of a plethora of "new" therapies, some more esoteric and unusual than others. These include such things as aromatherapy, reflexology, body therapies such as Feldenkrais, pulsing, Alexander technique, gem therapy, color therapy, Reiki, etc. You can contact any of the organizations listed in this chapter for more information about the therapies discussed.

Acupuncture

Acupuncture has a history stretching back 3500 years. First developed in ancient China, the practice spread into other Asian countries and was first introduced into Europe in the eighteenth century. Interest in its use in the United States was sparked as a direct result of former President Richard Nixon's trip to China in 1970, when an emergency operation was performed on a member of Nixon's staff using acupuncture as the only method of anesthesia.

Study by the American medical establishment followed, and today, after more than 20 years of clinical usage, acupuncture is used to treat a wide range of physical problems. There are currently more than 30 schools of acupuncture in existence in the United States, and around a dozen master's programs accredited by the National Accreditation Commission for Schools and Colleges of Acupuncture and Oriental Medicine in Washington, D.C. Admission requirements normally include courses in anatomy and physiology or other Western sciences, and the degree program usually lasts from three to four years.

The regulation and licensing of health care professionals differ from state to state throughout the United States, and the state laws regulating acupuncture vary widely. Some states do not regulate the practice, while in still others acupuncture can only be performed under the supervision of a licensed physician. Common credentials for individuals who are licensed or certified to practice acupuncture include the titles of Certified Acupuncturist (CA), Licensed Acupuncturist (LAc or Lic Ac), Master of Acupuncture (MAc), and Registered Acupuncturist (RAc).

For more information about professional standards and licensing requirements for acupuncturists, contact:

National Commission on the Certification of Acupuncture
1424 16th Street N.W., Suite 501
Washington, D.C. 20036
(202) 232-1404

The American Association of Acupuncture and Oriental Medicine, which shares the same address, provides referrals for practicing acupuncturists. Call (202) 265-2287 for more information.

How Does Acupuncture Work?

The answer is, no one really knows exactly! If you ask a Western medical acupuncturist this question, the answer will include talk of endorphins, neurons, and the parasympathetic nervous system.

Ask the same question of a traditional Chinese acupuncturist and you will hear of chi, energy, blood, meridians, and zangfu (internal organs).

Your body is traversed by a system of invisible energy pathways called meridians. This network of channels is the route along which energy, or chi, passes from one organ to another. There are 14 main meridians, 12 of which relate to internal organs. While the chi flows freely along the meridians, and in the right quality and quantity, you stay healthy. Ill health occurs when the chi flow is blocked, or becomes deficient or excessive in some way. This can happen as a result of poor living, emotional stress, environmental stress (such as exposure to cold, wind, and damp), dietary indiscretion, or as a result of constitutional weaknesses. Balance is reestablished through the use of acupuncture and moxibustion (an herbal complement to acupuncture therapy). By inserting fine needles at certain points along the meridian, chi can be drawn to that meridian (if the energy is deficient), or dispersed away from that meridian (if the energy is excessive).

Yin and Yang

Yin and yang theory is one of the main theoretical systems forming the basis of traditional Chinese acupuncture. This system is used to understand and describe the workings of the body (and at a much broader level, to understand the workings of the world in general). Chi (or energy or life force) is a composite of two opposing, interrelated energies labeled yin and yang. All things are seen as being made up of these two interdependent energies. Yang energy is represented by warmth, movement, expansion, dryness, hardness, and maleness. Yin energy is the more feminine, quiet, stilling, cooling, soft, and moistening energy. Thus in the world in general, nighttime is more yin than daytime; the spring is more yang than the autumn; the sunny side of the street is more yang than the shaded side! Yin and yang exist as equals—neither one is superior to the other. They each need the other to exist themselves, because they are both relative, rather than absolute, concepts. Something can only be considered yin in relation to something else—there is no such thing as absolute yin.

Within your body yin and yang energies are in a state of constant flux, depending on the time of day, the season, the stage of your menstrual cycle, etc. Should this flux become disturbed in some way, and either yin or yang energy become excessively strong or abnormally weak, the flow of your chi is disturbed, with the end result of ill health.

How Does the Acupuncturist Decide What the Energy Imbalances Are?

If you go to a traditional Western doctor with an illness, he or she relies upon a learned catalogue of symptoms of illness to make a probable diagnosis. Frequently the diagnosis will be confirmed through laboratory tests, such as urine or blood tests. When you go to a traditional Chinese acupuncturist, the diagnosing begins as soon as you take your seat in the waiting room. The way you walk, the color and amount of your clothing, your confidence or hesitancy, the tone and volume of your voice, the color of your face, and your physical build are all useful clues observed by your acupuncturist. The final diagnosis of your complaint is based upon the results of four main methods of diagnosis. These include:

- Looking

- Listening

- Asking

- Touching.

Looking involves noticing all the things described above in the waiting room scene, in addition to observation of facial color, complexion, signs of swellings, or other superficial abnormalities.

Your acupuncturist listens to discern any obvious features of your speech. Do you shout or talk very quietly? Does your voice have a laughing quality to it? Do you sigh a lot, or talk non-stop? Just as is the case with your trip to the doctor's office, an important part of the information-gathering involves a thorough case history.

Questions about your appetite, energy levels, thirst, bowel movements, urine, sleep, perspiration, and menstrual cycles will also be asked.

Finally, diagnosis through touching involves feeling the area of the body where your problem is occurring: looking for areas of abnormal heat or cold, or areas painful to the touch. One of the most important methods of diagnosis, unique to traditional Chinese medicine, is the taking of the pulses.

Pulse Diagnosis

Your acupuncturist will feel 12 pulses near your wrist. There are three pulse positions on each wrist, with a superficial and a deep pulse at each position. These pulses give your practitioner a clear picture of the condition of your chi flowing through your energy meridians. Each pulse position corresponds to one of the 12 internal organs, giving the practitioner a detailed insight into how your energetic imbalances are affecting individual organs and meridians.

And Now to Your Treatment

Using all the information gathered, the acupuncturist now formulates a plan of treatment tailored exactly to suit your particular imbalances. He or she will use acupuncture needles, and sometimes moxibustion as well, to rebalance the flow of chi through your energy meridians.

Acupuncture needles are usually made of stainless steel. They are extremely fine—sometimes barely thicker than a hair. The needles are solid, unlike the hollow hypodermic needles that are used for giving injections. If you have a fear of injections, do rest assured that acupuncture needles in no way resemble these hollow, thick, and painful hypodermic needles. Once inserted, the needles are usually left in place for about 20 minutes.

Moxibustion is used whenever your illness is the result of a weakness of yang (warming, active) energy. For example, if you exhibit symptoms of a weakness of the warming energy of the kidneys, such as a tendency to feel the cold, low backache, and frequent urination, moxa will be used to warm your needles.

Moxa is made from densely rolled dried mugwort herb. The moxa most commonly used is rolled in a long cigar shape. Your acupuncturist will hold the lighted cigar above certain needles to increase the yang chi in the affected meridians. Besides the strange-smelling smoke, having moxa is a very relaxing and pleasant experience. Sometimes small wedges of moxa are attached to the end of the needle itself.

The Question of Sterility

If you have acupuncture from a registered practitioner, you need have no worries about the sterility and safety of the acupuncture needles used. Sterilization procedures for reusable needles are regulated by state and federal agencies. All needles are pre-soaked in a potent anti-bacterial solution before undergoing sterilization in an autoclave of the type used to sterilize hospital surgical instruments. Most practitioners also offer their patients the option of disposable needles. These pre-sterilized needles are used only once before being safely disposed.

More and more Americans are aware of the benefits of acupuncture for treating musculo-skeletal injuries. However, not so many know of the wide variety of illnesses that can be helped by this ancient therapy. The World Health Organization has formulated a list of illnesses that have been proven to be effectively treated by acupuncture.

- Respiratory disorders such as asthma, bronchitis, and emphysema

- Skin disorders such as acne, eczema, and psoriasis

- Ear, nose, and throat complaints including colds, flu, tinnitus, sinusitis, nerve deafness

- Gastrointestinal disorders such as nausea, gastric ulcers, colitis, constipation, spastic colon, diarrhea, and hemorrhoids

- Cardiovascular problems including high and low blood pressure, angina, palpitations, and poor circulation

- Gynecological and urinary tract problems such as cystitis, bedwetting, menstrual problems, PMS, infertility, and pain relief during childbirth

- Neurological problems such as headaches and migraine, tics and tremors, trigeminal neuralgia, shingles, sciatica, general neuralgias, and numbness

- Psychological disorders including anxiety, depression, insomnia, and nervous tension.

Medical Herbalism

Herbalists use the naturally occurring medicinal properties of plants to treat body imbalances causing symptoms of illness. Because many of the modern pharmacological wonder drugs are made using chemicals extracted from plants, you may think that medical herbalism and pharmacological medicine have much in common. However, the common ground ends there.

Pharmacological medicine searches the plant kingdom looking for "active ingredients" that can be extracted from plants, isolated from the other naturally occurring substances, and concentrated as a tablet or medicine. Commonly used drugs such as reserpine (to lower blood pressure), digoxin (to treat heart failure), and morphine (a powerful painkiller) are all made from plant extracts. Because these drugs are concentrated and isolated forms of the beneficial plant chemical, they can also be extremely toxic and dangerous.

The medical herbalist acknowledges and respects the intricate balance of interacting chemicals and buffers which occur naturally in plants and herbs. By using the whole herb rather than one or a few of its concentrated "active" chemicals, the herbalist is usually able to provide a more gentle, less toxic treatment (with far fewer, if any, side-effects!).

Herbalism and pharmacological drug treatment differ in another fundamental way. Drug therapy aims to combat a particular illness or symptom, with little consideration to the overall well-being of the patient. A good herbalist is interested in more than simply treating your presenting symptoms. He or she will delve deeply, looking for underlying weaknesses and trying to establish what weak links predisposed you to become ill in the first place. Having gained a clear insight into your unique pattern of weaknesses, the herbalist uses herbs to stimulate your body's inherent healing energies, rather than simply to mask your symptoms of sickness.

Herbal medicine is enjoying a resurgence in the United States, with health food shops stocked to the brim with various herbal tablets, dried herbs, and tinctures. It should be recognized, however, that although they are natural, some herbs can cause unpleasant reactions if used unwisely by the untrained lay person.

Medical Herbalism in the United States

If you have a chronic health problem that you want to treat with herbs, it is in your own best interest to consult with a qualified medical herbalist. Although herbalism is not a licensed method of treatment in the United States, herbal treatments are prescribed by a number of medical professionals, including regular M.D.s who practice holistic medicine, naturopaths, and acupuncturists. For more information about botanical remedies, you can contact the following organizations:

American Botanical Council
P.O. Box 201660
Austin, TX 78720
(512) 331-8868; (800) 373-7105

Herb Research Foundation
1007 Pearl Street, Suite 200
Boulder, CO 80302
(303) 449-2265

American Herbalist Guild
P.O. Box 1863
Soquel, CA 95073-1863
(408) 464-2441

Herb Society of America
9019 Kirtland Chardon Road
Mentor, OH 44060
(216) 256-0514

American Herb Association
P.O. Box 1673
Nevada City, CA 95959
(916) 265-9552

Homeopathy

More and more medicine cabinets contain various bottles of homeopathic remedies alongside the aspirin and the cold remedies. It is relatively easy for lay people to learn to use basic homeopathic remedies effectively to treat acute problems such as burns, cuts, bruises, sprains, teething pain, etc. Most health shops carry homeopathic first-aid kits that come complete with easy-to-follow guide books for dealing with minor acute problems. It should be noted, however, that homeopathy is a very precise healing science, and its efficacy is directly related to the skill and accuracy of the prescribing homeopath. Results will only occur when exactly the right remedy is prescribed. For this reason, it is important that you seek professional homeopathic consultation when dealing with anything more than acute first-aid-type problems.

What Is Homeopathy?

A German medical doctor by the name of Samuel Hahnemann devised this system of healing in the late eighteenth century. Through personal experimentation with the anti-malaria drug quinine, Hahnemann found that a healthy person taking the drug would strangely exhibit some of the symptoms of malaria! With further experimenting, he came to realize that the supposed "symptoms" of the disease were features of the way the body mounted its self-defense against that particular disease. It followed then, that by giving a person with malaria tiny doses of quinine, the body's inherent healing ability would be stimulated.

Over a period of many years Hahnemann tested hundreds of the drugs of this time, giving small amounts of each to healthy volunteers called "provers." The "proved" remedies were then collated in a weighty tome known as the *Materia Medica*, which is still used by today's homeopaths.

Homeopathy Versus Allopathy

Homeopathy translates as "like disease," while allopathy (the system we recognize as modern Western medicine) literally means "opposite disease." A doctor gives you a medicine designed to produce the opposite symptoms to those you are complaining of. For example, if you complain of a fever, you are given anti-pyoretics such as aspirin to produce a state of non-fever and restore your temperature to normal. If you complain of the same fever to your homeopath, you will walk away with a remedy which, when given in large amounts to a healthy person, would cause them to develop exactly the symptoms of your type of fever! This philosophy of using "like to cure like" is one of the basic tenets of homeopathy.

Potentized Remedies

The second remarkable discovery to thank Hahnemann for is the realization that when a drug is diluted many times (even to the point where tests can find no traces of the original drug in the solution) it acquires even more dynamic healing abilities. The more dilute the remedy, the faster and more effectively it heals. This phenomenon only occurs when the diluted remedies are "potentized" by a vigorous shaking (known as succussion) after each dilution.

Any homeopathic remedy with a potency greater than 12 "c" (one part solution to 10^{24} parts alcohol or water) contains no trace of the original pharmacological agent it contained! This is one of the reasons why some "scientific" minds find homeopathy a difficult concept to accept. Clearly, this therapy operates on a much more subtle energetic level than traditional pharmacological medicine.

Preparing for a Visit to the Homeopath

Your first visit to a homeopath may be an unusual experience for you. Your practitioner uses a long process of detailed questioning to build up a clear picture of your exact symptoms, in order to choose the correct remedy. You will be asked to decide when your condition is worse and when it is better; whether it is affected by the time of day, the weather, noise, movement, eating, temperature, etc. There will probably be questions about your emotional makeup, your sleep and dreams, bowel movements, urine, appetite, thirst, energy levels, and a whole lot more as well.

Self-Help Homeopathy

Most health shops stock homeopathic remedies in the 30 c potency, suitable for treating acute conditions and injuries. This potency means that one part substance is added to 100 parts dilutant. This is succussed and then one part of this is taken and diluted with another 100 parts dilutant. This process is continued 30 times, to come up eventually with your 30 c remedy! When using these remedies there are some basic do's and don'ts you need to be aware of:

- Always store your remedies in a separate place from all your other medicines, perfumes, food, etc., as they will be detrimentally affected by strong smells. Preferably store them in an airtight container, in a cool, dark cupboard. Never put your remedy near linament, peppermints, or perfumes.
- Never touch the homeopathic remedy with your fingers. Shake tablets or pillules into the lid of the bottle before dropping them straight into your mouth. The tablets should be placed beneath your tongue and allowed to slowly dissolve. If you drop a tablet, throw it away.
- Take your remedy 15 minutes before or 30 minutes after food or drink.
- Try to avoid coffee, strong spices, peppermints, and mint chewing gum while using remedies.
- Don't use a strong-smelling vapor rub if you have a cold and are using homeopathic remedies at the same time. Use a homepathically friendly toothpaste made from all-natural ingredients, preferably without mint.

Naturopathy

The original "nature cure" naturopaths of old used the natural elements of fresh air, sunshine, and water (hydrotherapy), coupled with sound nutrition, regular exercise, and adequate relaxation, to stimulate and encourage the body's own innate healing abilities. Naturopaths teach the principles of balanced, healthy living to stay well. The emphasis of naturopathy is on staying well, rather than patching up the symptoms of ill health resulting from poor lifestyle habits. The naturopath's role is first and foremost as teacher and healthy living educator. Through teaching you how to live in accordance with nature's law, the naturopath provides you with the means to lead a healthier life.

Body, Mind, and Soul

As with other complementary therapies, naturopathy acknowledges that you are only as healthy as the sum total vitality of your body, mind, and soul. Physical health can only be achieved when spiritual, emotional, and mental health is present. Likewise, it is difficult to feel healthy emotionally if you are suffering the discomfort of a physical illness. When a naturopath treats you, the focus of attention is upon you and your wellness, rather than the symptom of ill health you are suffering from.

What Type of Treatment Will a Naturopath Prescribe?

Most naturopaths will advise you on changing many of the "wrong living" patterns that have made you sick in the first place. This may involve examining stressors and learning new ways to deal with them more appropriately; for example, through meditation or progressive relaxation. It will almost certainly involve detailed dietary analysis, followed by formulation of a new, more health-giving dietary regime for you to follow. There will probably be discussion about exercise, and recommendations for an appropriate physical program. These days many naturopaths will probably also send you away with a prescription for nutritional supplements, herbs, or homeopathic remedies, too.

Because your naturopath will not supply you with a magic bullet to take away your ills, you will need a fair degree of self-motivation, dedication, and perseverance to benefit from your visit. Naturopathic medicine is strong on self-responsibility and self-healing, but it is often very effective if you take the trouble to apply what you are taught.

Toxins

This is one of the naturopath's favorite words. Naturopathic medicine strongly believes in the concept of self-poisoning through a build-up of toxins in your body. These toxins arise from poor digestion, causing improper metabolism of proteins; poor liver function with resulting build-up of systemic poisons; constipation and absorption of toxins from the loaded bowel; and the daily addition of chemicals resulting from your "fight or flight" stress response.

These poisons literally pollute your body, hampering its normal physiological functions and making you look and feel less than well. Cleaning up your act usually involves supervised elimination diets or fasts; the use of colonics and enemas to cleanse the bowel; and frequent saunas and skin brushes to encourage the release of toxins through the skin.

Naturopathy in the United States

Naturopathy was introduced into the United States by Benedict Lust, who founded the American School of Naturopathy in New York City around the turn of the century. Although the discipline experienced a decline with the rise of pharmaceutical drugs after World War II, naturopathic practice has experienced a strong resurgence over the past 20 years.

John Bastyr College in Seattle; the National College of Naturopathic Medicine in Portland, Oregon; Ontario College of Naturopathic Medicine in Toronto; and the Southwest College of Naturopathic Medicine and Health Sciences in Scottsdale, Arizona, currently offer postgraduate programs leading to a Doctor of Naturopathy (N.D.) degree. Admission requirements match those of other medical schools, and the programs require four years of study in medical science along with training in naturopathic techniques.

Naturopaths are currently licensed in only seven states (Washington, Oregon, Arizona, Connecticut, Alaska, Hawaii, and Montana). Other states have either no regulations or a variety of specific rules governing practice. For more information or to locate practitioners close to you, contact:

American Association of Naturopathic Physicians
2366 Eastlake Avenue East
P.O. Box 20386
Seattle, WA 98102
(206) 323-7610

Osteopathy

In a little over one hundred years since its birth, osteopathy has become an important, respected, and widely used system of healing. In America, where it originated, osteopathy is a much respected branch of medicine, practiced by many medical doctors. There are large osteopathic hospitals where osteopathy is used in tandem with more traditional drug therapy. This proven therapy is now practiced around the world, with recognized training centers in America, Britain, and Australia.

Osteopathy literally means pathology (or sickness) of the bones. This manipulative medicine is concerned with the muscles, tendons, and connective tissues of the body as well as the skeleton. The basic premise of osteopathy is that structure governs function. Translated, this means that the healthy functioning of the body is dependent upon a sound structure. Misaligned bones (most especially the bones of the spine) and muscle spasms interfere with the nerve and blood supply to the tissues and vital organs of the body. Poor nerve innervation, reduced blood flow, and reduced oxygen supply eventually lead to degeneration and ill health. So, to an osteopath, that sore spot between your shoulder blades has more far-reaching implications than simply causing a little back pain. If left untreated, your spinal misalignment (or osteopathic lesion) may go on to become a chronic problem, eventually leading to more serious problems; for example, lung problems and asthma.

In common with all other complementary or holistic therapies, osteopaths recognize the body's basic self-healing abilities. They believe that this self-healing is hampered through structural musculo-skeletal imbalances, and by using osteopathy to realign the structure, the self-healing ability is maximized.

Osteopathy in the United States

Osteopathy was founded by an American doctor named Andrew Taylor Still in 1874. Dissatisfied with nineteenth century medicine and the use of drugs, Still went on to study the skeleton and tissues related to it to develop an alternative approach to diagnosis and healing. In its early days, the discipline's emphasis was on the spinal column. While the spine is still considered to be the most important part of the musculo-skeletal system, today's osteopaths are trained in the care of all the body's joints and muscles. If you injure an ankle, a knee, an elbow, or a shoulder, your osteopath is usually able to offer effective treatment.

Today, osteopathic physicians (Doctors of Osteopathy, or D.O.s) undergo training virtually indistinguishable from other doctors of medicine. There are presently 15 osteopathic medical colleges located throughout the United States, offering a four-year graduate-level curriculum of medical training, a one-year internship, and optional residency programs of from two to six years in a variety of medical specialities. While osteopaths are trained to take a holistic approach to treatment, they can also prescribe drugs, perform surgery, and draw on all of the other methods available to modern medicine. For referrals to the minority of osteopaths who rely on palpation or manipulation as their means of treatment, contact:

American Academy of Osteopathy
3500 DePauw Boulevard, Suite 1080
Indianapolis, IN 46268
(317) 879-1881

Even fewer practioners have been trained in cranial osteopathy. To find these psysicians, contact the Cranial Academy at the same address or by telephone at (317) 879-0713.

Cranial Osteopathy

Cranial osteopathy is one of the less well-known branches of osteopathic medicine in other Western countries, but in America, cranial is widely practiced, and is available in many hospitals. The maternity sections of American osteopathic hospitals all use cranial osteopathy as a matter of course on newborn babies.

The skull is not a rigid cage of bone. It is comprised of 29 bones knitted together with suture joints that allow the skull to move very slightly. During birth, a baby's skull bones are compressed and overlap each other, so its head can fit through the birth canal. Nature ensures that the baby's skull is flexible enough for this to happen. Unfortunately, this same flexibility can lead to problems for the baby in a complicated birth.

*How Do You Know If a Newborn Is in
Need of Cranial Osteopathy?*

If you had a difficult birth, and are now living with a cranky, irritable baby who is very difficult to settle; a baby with digestive problems such as colic, reflux, or any form of sleep disorder, you will probably both benefit from seeing a cranial osteopath.

Chiropractic

Chiropractic is the other main manipulative therapy, closely aligned with osteopathy. It had its evolution in America around the time that Andrew Taylor Still developed osteopathy. David Daniel Palmer, the founder of chiropractic, believed in a similar concept of structure governs function and the importance of structural integrity.

Chiropractors tend to place more emphasis upon modern technology when it comes to diagnosing a musculo-skeletal problem. Whereas an osteopath relies a great deal upon the sensitivity and skill of their hands to literally feel what the problem is, a chiropractor will nearly always insist on X-rays before treating a patient.

Like osteopaths, chiropractors use manipulation, in particular, spinal manipulation, to facilitate the body's natural healing ability. Most people seek the help of a chiropractor when they are suffering pain or limited movement of their back or neck.

While chiropractic and osteopathy have much in common, there are differences between the manipulative techniques used. Chiropractors tend to use less leverage in their adjustments, aiming more for a direct thrust against the particular offending vertebrae. Osteopaths, on the other hand, tend to use more soft tissue work (massage of various kind) before attempting an adjustment.

Chiropractic in the United States

Doctors of Chiropractic (D.C.s) undergo at least four years of a postgraduate program comparable in hours to medical school, with most accredited chiropractic colleges requiring around two years of college credits for admission. Chiropractors must pass written and oral examinations administered by national and state boards and are licensed by the state where they plan to practice. For additional information, contact:

American Chiropractic Association
1701 Clarendon Boulevard
Arlington, VA 22209
(703) 276-8800

Chapter 14

AIDS Awareness

As recently as the early 1990s, statistics seemingly supported the notion that AIDS was a disease affecting homosexual men and intravenous drug-users, and drug free heterosexual women could believe themselves safe. Today, the complacency has gone. AIDS is here to stay for the foreseeable future, and it is no longer confined to these two high-risk groups. HIV infection is now spreading faster among herterosexuals (both men and women) than among any other group.

HIV and AIDS

It is important to understand the difference between being HIV positive and having AIDS. You are declared HIV positive when you have a blood test that shows you have been infected with HIV (human immunodeficiency virus). Once you become HIV positive, there is a variable period of time during which there are no symptoms of ill health whatsoever. This latent period usually lasts somewhere between eight to 10 years, although in some it is substantially shorter.

AIDS (Acquired Immune Deficiency Syndrome) is the end stage of infection with HIV, in most cases. However, there are cases of HIV infection which have still not developed into AIDS 10 years after infection with the virus. Because this is such a young epidemic, it is still not clear if every case of HIV infection will eventually end with AIDS.

AIDS is the stage at which symptoms of infection with HIV become most severe. The immune system has been progressively weakened during the latent period of HIV infection, and now a host of infections and cancer overpower the weakened immune system. The HIV virus itself does not kill people, but infections such as pneumonia and various types of cancer, including the most common, Kaposi's sarcoma, do.

The following are some of the symptoms of late stages of HIV infection:

- Persistent headaches
- Dramatic weight loss for no explicable reason
- Swollen, painful lymph glands in the neck, underarm, and groin
- Deteriorating vision and spots before the eyes
- Persistent, dry cough
- Oral thrush (and vaginal thrush in women)
- Watery diarrhea
- Pain during bowel movements and rectal bleeding
- Night sweats.

HIV—A Hard Virus to Contract

Aids is the most feared epidemic of the day, and yet ignorance and misinformation still abound. HIV positive people are still discriminated against and needlessly feared. The truth is that the HIV virus is *not* easy to contract, provided you avoid high-risk activities such as unprotected sex with an infected partner, or sharing of hypodermic needles. The HIV virus is very weak, quickly dying outside the human body. It can be easily killed with ordinary-strength household disinfectant. HIV *cannot* be transmitted through ordinary body contact such as hugging, shaking hands, or even kissing. Sharing a cup, a telephone, a toilet, or a toothbrush with an infected person *will not* put you in any danger of contracting the virus.

HIV can only be transmitted from one person to another through an exchange of vaginal fluid, semen, or blood during sexual contact, or through skin piercing with a hypodermic needle or some other infected sharp instrument. HIV can also be passed on from an infected woman to her unborn baby during pregnancy or birth, but the maximum transmission rate from mother to baby is still only between 22 and 33 percent.

Putting Yourself at Risk

So what exactly are the high-risk behaviors?

- Sharing hypodermic needles.
- Having unprotected sexual intercourse (either vaginal or anal) or oral sex with an infected person. There are often tiny abrasions in the lining of the vagina and anus or on the penis, which allow the virus to penetrate into the bloodstream either from the vaginal fluid or semen. The risk is especially great if you have other sexually transmitted diseases (STDs), as these increase the likelihood of having sores or abrasions on the sex organs.

  Anal sex is acknowledged to be the most risky type of sexual practice when it comes to exposing yourself to HIV infection. The lining of the anus is partiularly prone to trauma during intercourse, as the walls of the anus are only a few cell layers thick.

HIV can also be transmitted during oral sex, as the semen and vaginal fluids can enter the bloodstream through cuts, sores, or gum abrasions in the mouth.

- HIV can also be transmitted through infected blood or blood products (although in the United States today all blood products are HIV screened). Tissue or organ donation, bone grafts, and semen donation can also transmit HIV.

Safe Sex

The terms AIDS and "safe sex" are inextricably linked in most people's minds. Safe sex is sex that reduces (but often does not completely eliminate) your likelihood of being exposed to HIV.

Safe sex is any sexual contact where there is no (or reduced) contact with genital secretions (semen and vaginal fluids)—kissing, cuddling, fondling, mutual masturbation, body rubbing, and sexual intercourse using condoms. Obviously sex becomes safer if you remain in a sexually exclusive relationship with an uninfected partner.

HIV and Women

Women as a group have been largely ignored in the research and publicity surrounding HIV and AIDS. This is partly a result of the original misconception that AIDS is a gay, male disease. One look at the facts and figures quickly dispels this fallacy. Today there are an estimated three million women infected with HIV throughout the world, and of these, 500,000 have already developed full-blown AIDS. In major cities in sub-Saharan Africa, western Europe, and the Americas, AIDS is now the leading cause of female death in the 20 to 40 years age group. HIV infection is increasing among women at an alarming rate. In the U.S., the 128,500 represented 11 percent of the total number infected in 1992—and the number of women with AIDS doubles every one to two years. Frightening statistics, aren't they?

Women are especially vulnerable to HIV infection through unprotected sexual intercourse, with a 12 times greater risk of infection than men. This is because in women there is a greater genital area (the mucosa, or lining, of the vagina), much of which cannot be seen and checked for abrasions or cuts. Having unprotected sexual intercourse during menstruation increases this risk even further. There is some concern that oral contraceptive pills may also increase vulnerability to infection, although this has not yet been conclusively proven.

There has been a lot of research into the effectiveness of various types of contraceptives in reducing incidence of HIV infection. The spermicide Nonoxynol-9 (available as cream and often used as a spermicide on condoms) has been shown to be deadly to the HIV virus, but there is also a high incidence of vaginal and cervical irritation when it is used frequently.

Female condoms, which are becoming readily available, also look to be a promising HIV-safe contraceptive. Fitted inside the vagina and held in place with a springy circular rim outside the vagina, the condoms are shown to be at least as safe as male condoms, and much more likely to be used by women unwilling (or unable) to ask their partners to take responsibility for contraception and safe sex.

AIDS in the United States

As of 1992, 1,167,000 people in the United States were infected by the HIV virus. Some 128,000 of these individuals are women. A total of some 328,000 cases were projected to occur in North America from 1992 to 1995 (with total cases throughout the world rising to 17,454,000 by 1995).

If you are worried that you may have been exposed to the HIV virus, you can be tested for HIV through your doctor, your local Sexually Transmitted Diseases Clinic, or at one of the AIDs centers.

Part Two

Getting Well

A-Z of Women's Health

Amenorrhea

Amenorrhea is the technical term to describe a lack of periods that cannot be explained by pregnancy or the menopause. Sometimes women stop menstruating without there being any other signs of ill health. Often, however, the lack of periods is simply part of an overall picture that includes exhaustion, anemia, or being underweight. There are two main categories of amenorrhea. Primary amenorrhea describes the 16- or 17-year-old teenager who for some reason has never started to menstruate. Secondary amenorrhea occurs when a woman who has had periods for years suddenly stops menstruating for no apparent reason.

Causes

If you miss the occasional period during times of great stress or when traveling, chances are you don't have much to worry about. Your monthly loss of blood is the end result of an intricate interaction between the brain, hormones, and your reproductive organs. This delicate balance is easily disturbed by stress, and once the stress eases, your periods will usually return. If, however, you have missed a period three or four times in a row, it's time to do some serious detective work.

Are you an exercise-aholic? Do you go to the gym at every opportunity, or consider a marathon a form of relaxation? The female body should carry a certain ratio of fat to muscle, and in these days of body image fixation, this ratio is often upset. If your percentage of body fat drops below 18 percent, your periods will probably stop. Ballet dancers, aerobic teachers, triathletes, and other fit sportswomen may go for years without menstruating. In the long run it can seriously affect their well-being.

Women with long-term amenorrhea have very low estrogen production, comparable with post-menopausal women. Estrogen protects your bones from demineralization. Without its calcium-sparing effects, your bones are prone to osteoporosis.

Crash dieting is another sadly common cause of amenorrhea. Trying to lose too much weight too quickly can leave your hormones knocked out of kilter, and unable to stimulate ovulation and menstruation.

A number of physiological disorders may be the cause of your lack of periods. These include diabetes, hyper- or hypothyroidism, hepatitis, Addison's disease, and Cushing's disease (the last two are adrenal gland disorders). However, your troubles are more probably due to less serious imbalances.

Perhaps you have recently come off the contraceptive pill? The pill causes profound changes in your hormonal balance, and the body is not always quick to reestablish its balance. Some women take months (or even years) to begin normal menstruation again after using the pill.

Your period is evidence of normal functioning and interrelation between the hypothalamus and pituitary gland (both parts of your brain), the thyroid and adrenal glands, and of course the ovaries and uterus. Problems in any one of these organs or glands can cause a cessation of periods.

It may be that your diet isn't all that it should be. Amenorrhea can be a direct result of malnutrition and anemia, resulting from frequent dieting, a poorly balanced vegetarian diet, or plain bad dietary habits. If you are anemic, you will possibly stop menstruating. Iron deficiency anemia is a very common problem among modern American women. Traditionally, iron was supplied by red meat and whole grains. With the trend to the reduction of red meat intake, and the move to white bread and refined cereals, iron deficiency has become increasingly common.

A lack of protein can also cause your periods to stop, although this is not especially common in the U.S., unless you exist on an imbalanced weight-loss diet.

So you see, there are a multitude of possible causes for your lack of periods. It is advisable to have a medical investigation to rule out serious physical problems before you embark on a self-help program.

Medical Treatment
This varies dramatically depending upon the cause of your problem, and may involve pharmacological treatment of an underlying condition such as diabetes or thyroid disorders. Where there is a clear psychological component, anti-depressants or tranquilizers are usually prescribed. Sometimes Clomiphene is prescribed to try to reestablish a normal cycle when the cause is thought to be hormonal imbalance.

Self-Help
If you've had all the tests and there is still no explanation for your lack of periods, maybe you need to take a good, close look at the quality of your existence. If you're living under a permanent load of almost intolerable stress, you need to find ways to diminish it, or at least learn new

ways of dealing with it, such as meditation, tai chi, or yoga. If your diet is erratic, unbalanced, and unhealthy, you need to do some serious reading (start with Chapter 2), and set about revolutionizing your dinner plate.

Look at your exercise regime. Do you exercise too much or not enough? Maybe you need to cut down on the aerobics and increase the yoga or meditation. If you're not exercising, begin a gentle program to stimulate your endocrine system and normalize your hormones. Simply going for a half-hour brisk walk three or four times a week will produce beneficial results.

Diet and Nutritional Supplements

Read the healthy diet outline in Chapter 2. Pay particular attention to your protein and fat intake. Too little dietary fat is usually only a problem if you are on a weight-reducing diet. Because fat is needed for the production of estrogen, make sure that you have some fat sources in your daily diet, preferably cold-pressed vegetable oils or oily fish.

A lack of B_6 and zinc are two of the most common findings in women inexplicably failing to menstruate. These deficiencies are especially likely to occur if you are on slimming diets, an unbalanced vegetarian diet, or a junk food diet (which probably accounts for a good 80 percent of women!). Read the B_6 and zinc sections in Chapter 2, and make an effort to include adequate dietary sources of these nutrients. Use supplementary sources as well—up to 100 mg of B_6 (along with a balanced B complex supplement) and 50 mg of elemental zinc each day. B_{12} and folic acid deficiency have also been implicated in the absence of periods, so if you are a strict vegetarian you may be lacking B_{12} (as well as protein).

It may be that your lack of periods is due to undiagnosed sluggishness of the thyroid gland (hypothyroidism). It is not uncommon for women to exist for years in a state of undiagnosed unwellness because of this problem. Ask your doctor for a thyroid function test if you are troubled by:

- Dry hair and skin, and thinning hair
- Excessive sensitivity to cold
- Poor immune function, and susceptibility to colds and infections
- Exhaustion and apathy
- Foggy thinking, inability to concentrate, depression, and anxiety
- Tendency to easy weight gain.

A Traditional Chinese Perspective

During the weeks following your period, your body refills your uterus with blood which then "spills over" at your next menstrual period. If the quantity and quality of your body's blood production is poor, there will be insufficient blood to refill your uterus. Consequently, there will be no "spilling over."

Most often, amenorrhea is the result of a deficiency of blood (that is, lack of quantity and quality), or from a stagnation of blood which impedes its flow. Traditional Chinese medicine considers the spleen and the kidneys to be the main organs involved with the body's production of blood. If either or both of these organs are weak, exhausted, and inefficient, the result can be blood deficiency. This weakness develops gradually from a variety of causes, including:

- Overwork, lack or relaxation, exhaustion, overindulgence in sex
- Ongoing emotional and physical stress
- Poor dietary habits: a lack of nourishment, excess of cold foods, eating at irregular times, and skipping meals.

Blood stagnates usually because of a weakness of chi (energy)—as chi is the force that moves the blood. Chi is weakened through "wrong living" as described above. Blood can also become stuck or stagnant due to the congealing effects of cold. The Chinese firmly advise against women exposing themselves to cold air or cold water before or during their periods. At this time the uterus is especially vulnerable to taking cold. Going for a swim in cool waters at this time would be most inadvisable.

The approach of traditional Chinese medicine to remedying amenorrhea involves the use of acupuncture and herbal formulas to tonify the blood by strengthening the kidney, spleen, and heart functions. Or, in the case of stagnation, to strengthen the flow of chi, and remove any cold blockage (through the use of the warming herb moxibustion). This kind of treatment is often extremely effective.

Hydrotherapy

A course of regular hydrotherapy can help to remove pelvic congestion and improve the health and functioning of your pelvic organs. To do this, alternate hot and cold sitz baths. Sit in a small tub of hot water, making sure that your bottom and lower abdomen are submerged, for no more than 10 minutes. Then repeat the process in another tub containing cold water. Stay in the cold tub for 30 seconds to a minute before returning to the hot tub. While you are sitting in the hot tub, have your feet dunked in the cold tub, and vice versa. Repeat this process three or four times. Sitz baths should be used two or three times a day for best results.

Herbal Help

Primary amenorrhea in adolescent girls can often be helped with a course of herbal uterine tonics such as blue cohosh, rue, false unicorn root, chasteberry, raspberry, and squaw vine. These same uterine tonics will help restore normal menstruation in women whose periods are delayed for some unknown reason. They are especially useful to restore a normal menstrual cycle in women who have recently come off the contraceptive pill. A useful uterine tea can be made up of two parts chasteberry, two parts false unicorn root, one part blue cohosh, and one part rue, to be drunk three times a day. Use one teaspoon of herbs to a cup of hot water.

The often used culinary herb sage is also useful to bring on delayed periods. Tincture of sage can be taken in doses of 50 drops twice a day until the period starts, at which time the dose can be reduced to 30 drops a day.

Homeopathy

- *Pulsatilla.* The type of amenorrhea treated by this remedy is usually accompanied by extreme emotional sensitivity and weepiness. There may be migraines and palpitations and a general sense of weakness. Often the periods have been suppressed by exposure to damp, such as in an excessively wet or humid climate or living in a damp house.

- *Dulcamara.* The periods have been suppressed through exposure to damp or cold. You are very sensitive to weather changes, which often result in colds or an attack of sinusitis. Your breasts often feel swollen and painful upon pressure.

- *Silcea.* This remedy can be used if your amenorrhea is accompanied by a tendency to feel the cold and in particular to have poor peripheral circulation. There is a general sensation of weakness and often constipation. There are usually skin complaints such as spots with pus or frequent boils.

In addition there are several homeopathic remedies that are clearly indicated if the exact cause of the cessation of menstruation is known. For example, if your periods stopped following your exposure to damp, Pulsatilla is indicated. If it was exposure to extreme cold or an emotional fright (fear), then Aconite is your remedy. Nat Mur is the remedy if your periods stopped following an emotional shock of some sort, while Ignatia is more specifically for grief.

Anemia

Iron Deficiency Anemia

By far the highest incidence of iron deficiency anemia is among women in their reproductive years. Anywhere between a quarter and a half of all menstruating women are found to have low reserves of the all-important mineral, iron. This is largely because of the regular monthly blood (and consequently iron) loss women experience as periods, and the drain on iron reserves experienced during pregnancy and lactation. During the later months of pregnancy a growing fetus demands 7 or 8 mg of iron a day—a large amount when you consider the average dietary intake to be only 15 to 25 mg a day. Poor dietary practices and frequent weight loss diets also take their toll on women's iron reserves.

Iron deficiency anemia does not occur overnight. It is the end result of months or even years of severe iron deficiency or excessive blood loss. It is possible (and quite common) to have low iron reserves and yet not display symptoms of anemia.

Diagnosis

This problem is officially diagnosed through blood tests specifically looking at your hemoglobin levels, hematocrit, and red blood cell count. The cells of your blood will also look abnormal beneath the microscope if you have iron deficiency anemia. The blood cells become smaller and paler than normal.

Red Blood Cell Count

It is your red blood cells that carry the red pigment (hemoglobin), which is responsible for transporting oxygen from your lungs to your tissues. If you have a low red blood cell count, this function cannot be performed adequately and you are considered anemic. A normal red blood cell count for an adult woman is about 4 to 5.5 million red blood cells in each cubic millimeter of blood.

Hemoglobin Level

This test determines the relative amount of oxygen-carrying pigment in your blood. Even if you have a normal red blood cell count, if your hemoglobin levels are low, you will exhibit symptoms of anemia.

In order for this hemoglobin to bind with the oxygen it transports to your tissue, it needs plentiful supplies of iron. This is why iron deficiency eventually leads to anemia. Normal hemoglobin levels are 12 to 16 gm per decilitre for women.

Ferritin Test

This test allows the cause of your anemia to be further differentiated. It provides the means of determining whether your anemia results from lack of iron or from chronic disease, inflammation, or infection. This test is a reliable gauge of iron stores.

Symptoms

What might prompt your blood tests in the first place is when you visit your doctor complaining of inexplicable lethargy or exhaustion. In menstruating women one of the first things to rule out, when these symptoms present, is anemia. If you have iron deficiency anemia, this lack of staying power results from a lower than normal number of red blood cells, low hemoglobin levels, and consequently poor oxygenation of your body.

As well as tiredness, you may also be complaining of headaches and dizziness, breathlessness, constipation, a poor appetite, and poor immune function with frequent infections. You may look pale and have a pale, sore tongue; your skin may itch for no apparent reason; and your nails may be brittle and break easily. Mental and emotional symptoms often also accompany anemia. These include apathy, irritability and depression, and possibly memory problems.

Causes of Iron Deficiency Anemia

The most obvious cause is a deficiency of dietary iron, and this occurs frequently in vegetarian women or those who spend their lives following one weight-loss regime after another. Your iron intake may be sufficient but you may have other dietary peculiarities which block the absorption of this iron. For example, drinking coffee or tea with or straight after your meals blocks iron absorption. A high intake of raw grains (such as cold cereals) supplies large amounts of phytic acid which combines with iron and pass it from the body in your stool. Taking large amounts of supplementary calcium can also block your absorption of iron.

Perhaps your problem is not poor iron supply, but poor absorption of the iron. If your stomach acid is low (hypochlorhydria), this mineral will remain largely unabsorbed and simply be passed from your body when you have a bowel movement.

Iron deficiency anemia can also result from a chronic loss of blood over many months, or from an acute trauma resulting in massive hemorrhaging. Undetected medical problems, such as a bleeding stomach ulcer, colitis causing intestinal bleeding, or even bleeding hemorrhoids, can all contribute to the development of anemia. If your menstrual periods are particularly heavy or long, perhaps because of undetected uterine fibroids, then you also run the risk of anemia. Even a normal period results in the loss of about 18 mg of iron, and about 10 percent of all women lose around 45 mg of iron due to their heavy bleeding.

Frequent use of some drugs can induce this type of anemia. These include the antibiotic tetracyclines (often prescribed for months on end to teenage girls for acne) and the commonly taken aspirin.

A low intake of vitamin C can lead to low iron reserves, as this vitamin is essential for the proper absorption of iron.

Treatment

If your doctor decides that you have iron deficiency anemia, you will most probably be given a course of iron tablets (usually ferrous gluconate, ferrous sulphate, or fumerate). While ferrous sulphate is an inexpensive and easily absorbed source of iron, it can also irritate your intestinal track, causing constipation and blackened stools. Ferrous gluconate and fumerate are also cheap and absorbable supplements and tend not to cause problems with constipation. If you are using these supplements, the recommended amount to take is around 325 mg two or three times daily. These high doses are specifically to treat anemia and shouldn't be used as a general preventative or ongoing supplement.

Other highly absorbable forms of iron include chelated iron such as iron aspartate and ferrous succinate. Whichever form of iron you end up using, you can further increase your absorption levels by taking a dose of vitamin C along with your iron supplement.

Iron supplements are not universally appropriate, and when taken in excessive amounts this mineral can cause a toxic syndrome called siderosis. The symptoms of "iron poisoning" include fatigue, loss of appetite and weight loss, headaches and nausea, vomiting, and shortness of breath. This overdose tends to be more of a concern in older people who are routinely prescribed iron tonics, and post-menopausal women who are no longer losing iron through menstruation. For growing children, menstruating women, and women during pregnancy and lactation, iron supplements in the region of 10 to 30 mg or iron a day are quite safe and often especially helpful.

Iron and Your Diet

Although iron occurs in a wide range of frequently eaten foods, not all dietary sources stand equal. There are two types of dietary iron—"heme" and "non-heme" iron. The heme iron is found in animal protein foods such as red meat, liver, and to a lesser extent chicken and fish. This type of iron is readily absorbed and utilized by your body.

Vegetarian iron sources such as grains, fruits, and vegetables contain the less readily absorbed non-heme iron. But there are ways you can enhance your absorption of this type of iron, either by eating it along with a little of the heme sources, or else by adding vitamin C-rich foods. Studies show that by adding as little as 60 mg of vitamin C to your non-heme meals, you can increase your iron absorption by 300 percent.

You can also increase your iron availability by decreasing your intake of iron-blocking foods at the time you are eating your iron-rich foods. In particular, this includes tea and coffee, and processed foods such as ice cream, soft drinks, cakes, cookies, and candies that contain phosphate food additives. (See the chart of pp. 60-61 for information on iron-rich foods.)

Other Types of Anemia

It is possible and quite common to exhibit all the signs of anemia, including the lab indicators of reduced numbers of red blood cells, while your iron status is perfect. An iron deficiency is by no means the only nutritional cause of anemia.

Deficiency of vitamins B$_6$, B$_{12}$, and B$_9$ (folate) can all induce anemia, as can zinc and vitamin E shortages.

If your hemoglobin levels fail to rise despite a lengthy course of iron supplements, the missing link could well be folate. This B vitamin found in grains and leafy green vegetables has been repeatedly found to boost hemoglobin levels when taken with iron in those women who failed to respond to iron alone. Folate is only of use to you if your B$_{12}$ status is normal. This vitamin (commonly lacking in strict vegetarians and elderly people with digestive problems) is essential for your body to change your dietary folate into a form it can utilize.

If your anemia fails to improve despite all these measures, see a nutritionally oriented health care professional for more detailed guidance and a solution to your health problem.

Cervical Dysplasia

If you are told that you have cervical dysplasia, don't panic and start thinking you have cancer. You don't. Dysplasia means abnormal cell development, in this case in the cells of your cervix. Cervical dysplasia is not a cancerous condition, although in some women it is a pre-cancerous condition. About 30 to 50 percent of women with cervical dysplasia will go on to develop cervical cancer, *if the condition is left untreated.* This progression usually takes from between three to seven years.

Cervical dysplasia, or CIN as it is referred to, is graded according to its severity, from grade 1 (mild and moderate changes) to grade 3 (most severe, and known as carcinoma in situ). Nobody knows exactly what causes cervical dysplasia but there are some factors that tend to be associate with its development.

One of these is sexual activity. If you started having sexual intercourse at an early age, and have had many different sexual partners, your risk of developing cervical dysplasia is greatly increased. It has been proposed that the sperm itself may cause abnormal cell changes when it comes into contact with the cervix.

Certainly women who use condoms or diaphragms for birth control have a lower incidence of dysplasia than women using the pill or an IUD. This would seem to be because the barrier methods prevent sperm from coming into contact with the cervix. There is some evidence that the hormones in the contraceptive pill may contribute to the development of cervical cancer. It has been shown that in women who develop dysplasia, those women who stay on the contraceptive pill are more likely to go on to develop cervical cancer than women who use another form of birth control. If you have been diagnosed with dysplasia, and you are using the contraceptive pill, it may be advisable to consider using a barrier contraceptive instead.

Certain viral diseases also increase your susceptibility to dysplasia. If you have genital herpes, or the genital wart virus, you fall into a high-risk group.

And What of Treatment?

If you have cervical dysplasia, your doctor will recommend some form of treatment to remove the abnormal cells. This will usually be performed through laser surgery or cryosurgery (where the cells are frozen off).

While removing the diseased cells is obviously a good idea, it makes sense also to address the question of why the dysplasia occurred in the first place. In clinical experiments one of the most common findings in women with dysplasia is the high incidence of nutritional deficiency. I would strongly advise any woman with dysplasia to take notice of this research and embark on an appropriate regime of nutritional supplements in the interest of preventing a recurrence of dysplasia. You should take advantage of the benefits of modern medical science and surgery, but at the same time take a close look at your lifestyle, diet, stress levels, and nutritional status.

Nutrition and Dysplasia

When it comes to preventing and treating dysplasia, the nutrients supreme are humble folic acid (part of the B complex of vitamins) and vitamin C. Folic acid alone has the power to heal even quite severe cases of dysplasia when taken in doses of 10 mg a day for about three months. Even if this treatment fails to cure the dysplasia, the folic acid dramatically reduces the likelihood of developing cancer of the cervix.

Women who take the contraceptive pill tend to have lower blood concentrations of folic acid than non-pills users. Read the information on folic acid in Chapter 2.

Whenever there is any kind of cell abnormality, or cancer, vitamin C is the first nutritional supplement to think of, and one of the most powerful immune function stimulants. Clinical studies have repeatedly shown women with dysplasia to have lower vitamin C intakes than women without dysplasia. Vitamin C should be taken with bioflavinoids, in several doses throughout the day, depending on bowel tolerance (see Chapter 2).

If your diet is lacking in the fat-soluble vitamin A, your chances of the dysplasia developing into cancer are greatly increased (by about 300 percent). This vitamin and its precursor form, beta-carotene, are vital for the healthy multiplication of cells in all the mucus membranes, including the vagina and cervix. Seek professional guidance before supplementing with large amounts of vitamin A, as it can be toxic. Alternatively, use the beta-carotene form of supplement, which can be safely taken in doses up to 100,000 iu a day without problems.

Preventing cancer involves a good deal more than swallowing a couple of vitamin pills each day. If you are serious about improving your health, you will need to change your diet—reducing saturated fats, refined carbohydrates, sugar, processed foods, and foods containing artificial preservatives and colors. You should also increase your intake of fresh (preferably organic) fruits and vegetables and vegetarian proteins (such as tofu, beans, and lentils). You would probably benefit from a period of detoxification, using colonic irrigation or enemas, and following a detoxification diet or fasting. You need to see a health care professional for guidance in this area.

Stress reduction, or at least learning how to remain unstressed by your stress, is also a vital part of your healing. Read Chapter 4 on relaxation and meditation, and read some of the further reading books mentioned in the appendix.

Other Ways of Helping Yourself

Many pelvic and gynecological problems have traditionally been helped by regular hydrotherapy (the use of water for healing), in this case in the form of alternating hot and cold sitz baths. This technique is discussed fully earlier in this chapter, and is most beneficial if performed two to three times daily.

Herbal pessaries made from cocoa butter and the powerful blood cleansing herb chaparral have traditionally been used for cervical and uterine problems. The anti-cancer herbs red clover and blue violet leaves can also be taken orally in the form of teas—30 grams of each herb to be added to one cup of water. It is in your best interest to seek professional advice from a registered medical herbalist if you want to use herbs to prevent the progression of your dysplasia.

In her book *Natural Healing in Gynecology*, Rina Nissim recommends the following preparation for use for dysplasia:

- Make a solution of 60 g of sweet almond oil, 20 g of wheat germ oil, 10 g of essential oil of thuja and 10 g of essential oil of cyprus.

- Soak a tampon in the solution and insert it high into the vagina, against the cervix.

- Use this solution every night before bed, and remove the tampon the following morning.

Chlamydia

Chlamydia is a sexually transmitted bacteria contracted through unprotected intercourse with an infected partner. Like Trichomonas, it is possible to become infected with chlamydia without there being any immediate symptoms. You may carry chlamydia for years, only becoming aware of it when you find that you are unable to conceive. If you have more than one sexual partner, are under 25 years old, and are using the contraceptive pill, your risk of contracting chlamydia is greatest. If you suspect that you may have this infection, it is vital that you get it treated quickly. The chlamydia bacteria can travel from the vagina up through the uterus, and along the fallopian tubes to the surrounding organs. This can cause pelvic inflammatory disease, and infertility.

Symptoms

There may be no symptoms of infection, or the symptoms may not appear for two weeks or up to seven months after infection. If you experience any of the following symptoms, you should see your doctor promptly, and ask to be tested for chlamydia:

- Lower abdominal pain, and deep internal pain during intercourse
- An urge to urinate frequently, and a burning pain when passing urine
- An unusual vaginal discharge.

Medical Treatment

Medical treatment is with powerful oral antibiotics such as tetracycline. Penicillin is useless against chlamydia. It is important to have your sexual partner tested and treated simultaneously, to reduce your chances of re-infection. During and after a course of antibiotics it is wise to consume large amounts of *Lactobacillus acidophilus* yogurt, to replace the "friendly" bacteria in the intestinal tract which are killed by the antibiotics. This will reduce your likelihood of stomach upsets and diarrhea caused by the drugs. You will also benefit from using yogurt-soaked tampons in the vagina. Replace the tampons two or three times daily. This greatly reduces your chances of developing a vaginal fungal infection as a result of the effect of the antibiotics upon your vaginal pH.

Cystitis

Do you rush to the toilet every 10 minutes, and still feel as though your bladder is full? Does your urine burn like fire water? If your answers are yes, the chances are you are suffering from a urinary tract infection, or cystitis. If you are a woman, you are many times more likely than your male partner to suffer from bladder infections. The reason is a purely structural one.

Bacteria finding their way from the outside world to the bladder in a male have six to eight inches of urethra to travel up. This compares to the tiny distance of about 1.5 inches in a female.

Once inside your bladder, these foreign bacteria (which are most commonly the *E. coli* bacteria often found living in the intestines) cause inflammation and irritation to the bladder tissues.

Symptoms

The most usual symptoms of cystitis include:

- Frequent urge to urinate, night and day

- Sensation that the bladder is never empty, even after passing water

- Burning sensation when voiding

- Pain just above the pubic bone or in the lower back.

Causes

There are a number of traditionally acknowledged causes of cystisis, such as those discussed here. However, it seems sensible to ask why, if these are the "causes" of cystitis, don't all women fall prey to constant urinary tract infections? How come there are many women in the world who never experience a bladder infection?

The answer surely lies in differing individual levels of health and immunity. Cystitis is an infection, and as with all infections, those with poor nutritional status, poor cellular health, and ineffective immune systems will be much more susceptible to its threat. Women do not all develop a case of cystitis each time a stray *E. coli* bacteria finds its way up to the bladder. As is the case with many of the other genito-urinary infections, it is common to play host to potentially unfriendly bacteria for weeks, months, or even a lifetime without them causing any health problems at all. It is only when the overall health of the whole body is reduced (for example, through a period of great stress such as a divorce or the death of a loved one) that the bacteria are able to undergo a population explosion.

If you suffer from more than the occasional bout of cystitis, you need to focus on increasing your level of total well-being through lifestyle and dietary changes. This will be more effective in reducing your number of cystitis attacks than spending your life avoiding sources of infection.

So, What Are the Traditionally Accepted Causes of Cystitis?

Since *E. coli* bacteria normally live in the bowel, incorrect toilet procedure can transfer the bacteria to the vagina or urethra. After a bowel movement, always wipe away from, rather than toward, your vagina. This is important, too, if you suffer from frequent attacks of vaginal thrush, as the *Candida* fungal spores often exist in the bowel. *E. coli* can also be transferred from the bowel if your partner touches your anus with any body part, and then goes on to touch your clitoris or vagina during lovemaking.

With even the best of hygiene, the act of sexual intercourse can be followed 36 hours later with an attack of cystitis. The thrusting motion of the penis, combined with the tiny distance from the outside world to the female bladder, enables bacteria to be literally pushed up toward the bladder. This is particularly likely in the traditional missionary position of intercourse.

If your pelvic floor muscles are weak, your bladder may prolapse and bulge forward into the wall of your vagina. If the back part of the bladder droops below the neck of the bladder, it becomes virtually impossible to empty your bladder properly (a bit like peeing uphill!), leaving an almost permanent reservoir of urine in your bladder. This stagnant urine provides a haven for bacteria to multiply and irritate the bladder.

What goes in one end of the body must come out the other end. An overdose of hot spices, coffee, and alcohol can cause irritation to the delicate tissues lining your bladder and urethra. There are also other less conventionally accepted factors that may be the cause of your chronic cystitis problem.

Waste materials are excreted from your body through several different channels:

- The bowel in the form of feces
- The lungs in the form of carbon dioxide
- The skin in the form of perspiration
- The kidneys and bladder in the form of urine.

If any one (or several) of these "garbage disposals" is lazy, it places an excessive load on the others. If you only manage a half-hearted bowel movement every two or three days, you are placing an undue load on your kidneys and bladder as accumulated toxins are passed out this way instead. So in this sense there is a direct link between constipation and cystitis!

The abdomens of children and teenagers house a variety of organs, each tidily tucked in their designated position. Unfortunately, having children, growing older, carrying a spare tire of fat, poor posture, and spinal problems all conspire to wreck this perfection. All this can cause the large part of the colon which lies across the abdomen from right to left (the transverse colon) to sag in the middle. This sagging weight in turn squashes and compresses all the organs beneath it, including the bladder. Blood flow is impeded and the long-term result is congestion and a downgrading of tissue health.

A bladder starved of oxygen and nutrients is a bladder ripe for infection. This same kind of poor tissue health can occur as a direct result of chronic spinal problems. All your pelvic organs receive nerve impulses from the spine. A back problem anywhere from shoulder-level down to the coccyx (tail bone) can affect the health of the bladder. In fact, I have personally seen cases of acute cystitis fixed almost overnight, following spinal manipulation from an osteopath.

Medical Treatment

The medical treatment of simple acute cystitis is a course of antibiotics from 1 to 10 days in duration. Relapses within a couple of weeks are common, and may be due to the initial offending bacteria not being completely overcome by the antibiotics. With what you now know, you can understand that there are a multitude of deeper, more constitutional reasons for cystitis than simply an invading bacteria. Consequently, simply shooting at the bacteria, while ignoring the health of the rest of the body, is like putting a plaster cast on an amputated limb.

Self-Help Treatment

Long-term preventative changes make a lot more sense than using natural remedies time and time again to deal with the symptoms of acute cystitis. If you want to prevent another case of cystitis, follow these precautions:

- Wipe from front to back after a bowel movement.

- Change pads and tampons frequently during a period.

- Encourage your partner to wash thoroughly before sexual contact, and try to avoid the transfer of bacteria from the anus to the vagina during sex play.

- Avoid tight-fitting jeans, and nylon pants and tights. Cotton pants and crotchless tights or stockings and suspenders allow more air flow and ventilation.

- Make a habit of drinking more water, rather than tea or coffee. Aim for seven or eight glasses of water a day. This keeps your urine diluted and less favorable to bacteria. It also keeps the urine flowing frequently, thus washing out any problematic bacteria.

- Make a habit of emptying your bladder frequently. Women who ignore their urge to urinate and hold on for long periods of time are more likely to develop cystitis. When you need to go, go right away!

- Get into the habit of getting up to pass water soon after sexual intercourse. This will help to wash out any bacteria that may have been pushed up the urethra.

- See a registered osteopath or chiropractor if you think you may have spinal problems that may be contributing to recurring cystitis.

- Eat wisely, exercise regularly, and relax frequently—in short, follow the guidelines for healthy living in the Chapters 2, 3, and 4 of this book!

- Follow the "immune booster" nutritional program outlined on p. 58.

Self-Help for Acute Cystitis

So you have promised yourself you will make all the long-term changes, but now you're in agony and you want some fast action. What can you do? Start drinking lots. Stay away from tea, coffee, and alcohol, and drink plenty of water, parsley tea (which will really get you running to the toilet), and cranberry juice. Try to find unsweetened cranberry juice, or cranberry juice sweetened with other fruits only. In a pinch, Celestial Seasons Cranberry Cove tea can be a substitute. The cranberries change the pH of your urine, making it more acidic and less hospitable to bacteria. Have four or five cups of strong cranberry juice or tea a day. If you can't get hold of cranberry juice or the tea, try drinking buttermilk (acidophilus), or a glass of water with two teaspoons of apple cider vinegar—they all perform the same acidifying function.

Change your diet to acidify your urine, too. While you have an acute attack, eat plenty of acidic foods such as grains, nuts, seeds, fish, dairy products, meat, and bread. Cut back on fruit and vegetables. (This way of eating is not a good idea long term—just for a few days.)

If your urine stings you when you void, try sitting in a bowl of warm water to urinate, or spray your vulva with warm water as you pass water.

Nutritional Supplements

Increase your vitamin C intake up to your bowel tolerance, with repeated doses every two hours. Because you are fighting an infection, your vitamin C tolerance will probably be very high. You may find that you can take 10 to 15 g over a 12-hour period without it causing diarrhea. Vitamin A (such as halibut liver oil capsules) can be increased to 30,000 iu a day—that is, three capsules, twice daily. If you are pregnant, don't use this vitamin without professional guidance.

A high potency B complex supplement is also a good idea while you fight the infection, and should be taken twice daily, with food.

Herbs

Many herbs can be used as urinary antiseptics. These include buchu, golden-seal, juniper berries, and garlic. Demulscents are herbs that soothe inflamed mucous membranes (such as the inside of the bladder and the urethra). These include such herbs as marshmallow root, couchgrass, and cornsilk.

An old naturopathic cure for burning urine involves mixing together equal parts of fennel, burdock, and slippery elm. Steep a teaspoon of this mixture in a cup of boiling water for 20 minutes. Drink when cold, one cup before each meal and then again before bed.

Two herbal teas for cystitis are particularly effective. They are flax-seed tea and a tea made up of equal parts of uva ursi and buchu. Make the teas using 1 teaspoon of dried herbs to a cup of boiling water. Allow to steep for 15 to 20 minutes, and drink one cup three or four times a day.

Homeopathy

- *Cantharis*. For cystitis characterized by frequent, painful, and burning urination, accompanied by violent spasms of shooting pain. This is the best remedy for the majority of cystitis cases.

- *Causticum*. For chronic cystitis accompanied by loss of bladder control.

- *Sarsparailla*. For cystitis with pain that is worse on completing urination.

- *Mercurius*. For classic cystitis with a frequent urge to urinate, burning urine, and dark urine passed in small amounts. The pain is worse when not passing water, or at the start or finish of urination. All the symptoms are worse at night.

- *Nux Vomica*. For burning or pressing pain during urination. Cystitis accompanied by extreme irritability and bad temper.

- *Apis*. For burning urine with a strong urge to urinate, but the ability to pass only a small amount of urine. Abdomen is very sensitive to pressure.

- *Arsenicum Alb*. For acute cystitis with burning pain and frequent urge to urinate. Symptoms are relieved by heat or warmth, for example, the application of a hot water bottle.

- *Pulsatilla*. Indicated more for mild but chronic cystitis. The patient is usually thirstless, and cannot stand any kind of heat.

Hydrotherapy

Traditional hydrotherapy for cystitis involved the use of hot sitz baths or hot compresses over the bladder. Simply dip a small hand towel in a basin of water as hot as you can bear. Ring out and quickly apply to the area just above your pubic bone. Repeat the process as the cloth cools, applying the compress eight or nine times, on two or three occasions throughout the day.

For a sitz bath, fill a small tub with water as hot as you can bear. Add five or six drops of bergamot oil to the water. Sit so the water covers your pelvis and lower abdomen for half an hour. Keep replenishing with fresh hot water to maintain an even temperature. Do not use hot sitz baths if you have a weak heart or high blood pressure.

Aromatherapy

Bergamot oil is most effective for treating cystitis. Take a couple of drops diluted in a tiny amount of honey. Repeat twice daily.

Packs

A hot water bottle over the lower abdomen and another over the lower back will help any aching pains.

Acupuncture

Acupuncture can be useful during an acute attack of cystitis. It is also an effective therapy to rectify the deep-seated imbalances that may be predisposing you to recurring attacks of cystitis.

Traditional Chinese Medicine

Traditional Chinese medicine views cystitis as being the result of an accumulation of damp and heat in the bladder. Treatment of acute cystitis aims to clear the damp and heat, using points on the lower abdomen, lower legs, and arms. Long-term treatment aims to stengthen underlying weaknesses. Frequently spleen and liver imbalances are part of the underlying problem.

Dysmenorrhea/Period Pain

In the western world, dysmenorrhea is one of the most common causes of lost work and school hours for women. Of 75 million women who menstruate in America, nearly half have menstrual pain regularly. Three and a half million of these women are completely incapacitated for one to two days every month because of pain.

Symptoms

You may experience lower abdominal and lower back pain, which can range from a dull, heavy ache to severe cramping similar to labor pains. There may also be diarrhea and vomiting.

Causes

There are two main classifications of dysmenorrhea—primary and secondary. Primary dysmenorrhea usually begins within the first few years of menstruation. Gynecological examinations fail to find any kind of disease of the uterus. The cramps usually begin within a few hours before or after the bleeding begins. This is by far the most common type of period pain. The pain is the result of the uterus contracting (in much the same way as it does during childbirth) under the influence of a type of local hormone called a prostaglandin.

Secondary dysmenorrhea is the result of some organic abnormality of the uterus, such as endometriosis, fibroids, polyps, cancer, or the presence of an IUD. This syndrome tends to start with a dull aching in the abdomen, up to ten days before bleeding starts. This pain may go away when your period starts, or it may persist right to the end of the period.

So What Actually Causes the Pain?

In the 1930s a major breakthrough in the understanding of period pain came with the discovery of prostaglandins. These local hormones regulate the tone of smooth muscles such as the uterus, blood vessels, and intestines. The smooth muslces contract, depending on the type and amount of prostaglandins you produce.

The lining of the uterus produces prostaglandins E and F, with the highest concentration occurring when the menstrual bleeding starts. When the uterus produces too many prostaglandins, or when type F is produced in excess of type E, it causes the uterus to become overactive. It contracts excessively and causes cramping and the all-too-familiar pain.

The uterus is designed to carry and then expel a baby, and as such it is a very powerful muscle. During menstrual cramps it contracts so powerfully that it cuts off its own blood supply, by compressing the uterine blood vessels. When a muscle is deprived of oxygen in this way (as also occurs during an angina attack), the pain is excruciating.

Once they have wreaked havoc with your sanity, these same uterine prostaglandins can escape into the bloodstream and go on to affect other smooth muscles in your body. For example, the intestines may be over-stimulated and contract too quickly, causing diarrhea. The blood vessels may dilate and allow blood to pool in your legs and feet, which in turn deprives the brain of blood and oxygen, and may cause you to faint.

It's hard to imagine that so much suffering can be attributed to the effects of one tiny chemical imbalance, but this seems to be the case. Women who suffer from dysmenorrhea have five times as much prostaglandin in their menstrual blood as their non-suffering peers.

Medical Treatment

If your doctor diagnoses primary period pain, he or she may well recomend the contraceptive pill. By preventing ovulation, the pill changes your hormonal balance and prostaglandin production and usually results in pain-free periods (which are not really periods, just withdrawal bleeding).

If you don't want to take the pill (or can't because you fall in the high-risk category), you will probably be prescribed some type of pain-killing drug, such as aspirin. Aspirin belongs to a group of drugs called "non-steroidal anti-inflammatories." These drugs appear to help period pain by slowing down or stopping the production of prostaglandins in the uterus, and consequently reducing the hard contractions.

A drug called mefenamic acid, which is sold over-the-counter in Austrailia and New Zealand, is available with a doctor's prescription in the U.S. under the brand name Ponstel. It inhibits prostaglandins in the same way as aspirin. Some users report symptoms of nausea, diarrhea, and indigestion. It is not suitable for asthmatics.

Nutrition

It is possible to reduce or eliminate your period pain without having to resort to drugs. When it comes to nutrition, the most effective treatment involves using therapeutic doses of the minerals calcium and magnesium.

Magnesium

Magnesium deficiency is common among women in areas with mineral depleted soil, and especially so in those who consume a high-meat diet, or who take calcium supplements that are not balanced with magnesium. Common signs of deficiency include muscle cramps, feelings of anxiety and depression, and twitching muscles and eyelids. Magnesium has been used successfully to relieve the misery of menstrual cramps. Read how to use magnesium in Chapter 2 on nutrition.

Calcium

Calcium is nature's painkiller. It greatly increases women's pain tolerance. Like magnesium, calcium is often lacking in diets, and it is not particularly effectively absorbed by the body. Calcium and magnesium are best taken in combination in a balanced formula supplying twice as much calcium as magnesium.

During acute menstrual cramps you can take a calcium and magnesium supplement as frequently as every 15 minutes, for three or four doses until your cramps subside.

Aspirin and mefenamic acid are both pharmacological prostaglandin inhibitors. Nature's version of the same is simple vitamin E. As well as inhibiting these pain-causing chemicals, vitamin E increases blood circulation and increases the amount of blood carrying oxygen to the uterus.

It is suspected that the cutting off of oxygen to the muscles of the uterus during a contraction is partly responsible for the cramping pain. As little as 100 iu of vitamin E taken daily throughout your cycle can reduce your period pain. On your painful days you can increase your dose to 400 or 500 iu, as long as there are no contraindications (see Chapter 2).

Essential Fatty Acids and Period Pain

The prostaglandins that cause the uterus muscles to contract are not the whole story. Your uterus also produces PGE 1 prostaglandins, which inhibit cramping. Not all prostaglandins are bad when it comes to period pain

Your body uses different raw materials to produce the different types of prostaglandins. Those prostaglandins that contribute to excessive cramping are manufactured from a substance that you ingest through animal fats such as meat, butter, and lard. The "anti-cramping" PGE 1 prostaglandins are manufactured by your body using the raw materials provided by vegetable oils such as linseed, borage, and evening primrose oils.

You can manipulate your body's production of these prostaglandins by decreasing the raw materials used to form the "cramping" prostaglandins and increasing your intake of the raw materials needed to make the "relaxing" PGE 1 prostaglandins. Cut out all animal fats, increase your intake of cold-pressed vegetable oils, and take evening primrose oil supplements (two 500 mg capsules, three times a day throughout your cycle).

Herbal Help

Several helpful herbs are traditionally used for this problem. "Women's" herbs such as raspberry leaf, squaw vine, cramp bark, and blue cohosh have provided relief for women for hundreds of years. Simply making raspberry leaf tea a part of your everyday diet may help you. This herb is a wonderful hormonal regulator and also a uterine tonic. Alternatively, why not try a strong brew of chamomile tea when you are in pain? Chamomile is an effective relaxant, and soothes cramping pain.

You can also make up your own herbal teas using dried herbs purchased from an herbalist (or available from some health food stores). If your cramping accompanies normal or heavy bleeding, try making a tea using the anti-spasmodic herbs black haw and cramp bark. Measure around half an ounce of each into a china teapot, and pour into one cup of boiling water. Leave the tea to sit for around 10 minutes before straining and drinking.

If your blood loss is scanty and accompanied by pain, you can use black cohosh and blue cohosh to make your tea. Follow the same procedure as above, using a quarter-ounce pinch of each herb. These herbs will encourage menstrual flow, and at the same time lessen cramping pain due to their analgesic (painkilling) chemicals.

Hydrotherapy

Hot sitz baths have been used for hundreds of years to ease the misery of menstruating women. Fill a small tub with hot water (about 100 degrees) and submerge your bottom and lower abdomen for about half an hour. Keep topping up with hot water to maintain a regular temperature. You can try adding herbal infusions or a few drops of essential oil to the water to enhance its effect.

A strong brew of chamomile tea or lemon balm tea will both help relax you and lessen the cramps. Five or six drops of essential oil of marjoram or rosemary could be added instead.

Homeopathy

In order to use homeopathy to treat your period pain effectively, you must determine the exact timing and nature of your pain so that the correct remedy can be selected. First, does your pain occur mostly before you begin bleeding? If it does, you will probably find your remedy in the following group:

- *Belladonna.* The face is usually flushed red. There is great sensitivity to any kind of movement or touch, which makes the period pain worse. The pain feels like a very heavy dragging sensation in the lower abdomen and pelvis.

- *Calcarea.* The pain is often accompanied by a sensation of weakness and general unwellness and nausea. The pains are colicky and often accompanied by noticeable sweating.

- *Chamomilla.* Great emotional sensitivity, with a sense of great anger and intolerance of noise or other people. Pain is severe and colicky before the onset of bleeding. This may be accompanied by vomiting, diarrhea, and fainting.

Another group of remedies is indicated if your pain occurs once your menstrual period actually begins:

- *China.* This remedy is indicated when the periods are heavy and clotty, and often early. Along with the low abdominal cramping, colicky pains, there is a feeling of great exhaustion, sometimes to the point of collapse.

- *Graphites.* Again the pain is sharp and cramping, but often it is in the lower back, and is accompanied by nausea, generalized body aches and chest pain.

- *Nux Vomica.* This type of pain is more in the lower back, and accompanied by constipation but with an urge to urinate frequently. There is often nausea and a very irritable and angry disposition.

- *Phosphorus.* There are a lot of emotional symptoms with this remedy. The sever contraction-like pains felt in the back are accompanied by anxiety and fearfulness. Headaches and an inability to get warm also accompany the pain.

Exercise and Period Pain

Regular exercise, throughout the month and while you are menstruating, can make a dramatic difference in your period pain. Exercise improves blood circulation, increases the oxygenation of your cells (including those in your pelvis and uterus), and generally assists in decongesting the pelvic area. A brisk walk three or four times a week may be all that you need to lessen or eliminate menstrual cramps. Stretching exercises are all useful, particularly those that stretch the loser abdomen and lower back.

Massage

Acupressure and massage are very useful tools to cope with period pain. Firm massage to the lower back and sacrum area will help to decongest the uterus. Using a little oil, ask your partner to press and rub either side of the spine and over the sacrum (the triangular-shaped bone at the bottom of the spine), for 10 minutes or so. The relief is wonderful. The following acupressure points are also useful:

- *Spleen 6.* On the inside of the lower leg. The point is four finger widths above your inside ankle bone. The point is found just behind your shin bone.

- *CV4.* This point is found on the lower abdomen. Find the halfway point between the navel and the crest of your public bone. Now move down about one inch from this point. This is the level of CV4, and the point lies exactly on the midline of the abdomen.

- *Spleen 8.* On the inside of the lower leg. The point is one and a half hand widths below the knee crease. The point is found just behind your shin bone.

Acupuncture and Osteopathy

If all the self-help procedures fail to make a difference in your monthly misery, you may well find more effective help from a professional acupuncturist or osteopath. Your uterus receives nerve impulses from the spinal nerves which emerge from the lower vertebrae of your spine. If you have a lower back problem (which you may not even be aware of), these spinal nerves are impinged, blood circulation and lymph drainage in you pelvis is reduced, and over a period of years the health of your uterus dimishes. A few visits to a registered osteopath or chiropractor for spinal manipulation may completely alleviate your menstrual problems.

Acupuncture is another traditionally effective therapy for all kinds of menstrual problems, including period pain. You will probably need several visits, both between and during your periods.

Endometriosis

Endometriosis affects between 10 and 15 percent of all menstruating women. Hundreds of thousands of women in the 25- to 45-year age group suffer the pain and infertility caused by this illness. Forty percent of all sufferers are unable to conceive.

Endometriosis can wreak its permanent damage in a sinisterly silent way. Months and years of gradual damage may have occurred before symptoms are considered unusual or severe enough to be investigated. Once symptoms do occur, it may be years (if ever) before the woman acknowledges she has a health problem and seeks help. Too many women are conditioned to accept period pain (which is one of the main symptoms of this disease) and a whole host of other "women's problems" as simply being their lot.

So What Is Endometriosis?

The lining of the uterus is called the endometrium. In a healthy woman, this lining gradually thickens between periods in preparation for receiving a fertilized egg. If this egg doesn't arrive in the womb, the blood-rich lining is sloughed off and travels out of the body as a menstrual period (see description of menstrual cycle, pp. 20-22).

Endometriosis occurs when stray fragments of the endometrium escape into the pelvic cavity and attack different pelvic organs. It is not known exactly how this occurs, but the most popular theory to date is that during a period, fragments of the uterus lining flow backwards up through the fallopian tubes and out into the pelvis. From here the stray tissues embed and grow on the ovaries, fallopian tubes, bladder, bowel, cervix, and the ligaments that hold the uterus in place. The most recent research, by Dr. David Redwine of Oregon, seems to indicate that these abnormal cells are present in the pelvic cavity from birth, making endometriosis a congenital condition. However, this is not yet the most widely recognized theory.

No matter how they get into the pelvic cavity, once there, these rogue cells behave as though they were still in the uterus. Thery are still controlled by the female sex hormones, and consequently mimic the plumping and sloughing cycle that is going on every month in your uterus. The blood that is released outside the uterus has no exit and simply settles and hardens on tissues in the pelvic cavity. The formation of scabs causes inflammation, and scar tissue eventually forms. At this point, a woman's fertility is greatly reduced. These misplaced endometrial tissues also have the ability to grow and spread to neighboring pelvic organs.

Symptoms

How do you know if you have this horrific-sounding disease? The main symptoms can be described in one word—pain. Be suspicious of periods that become painful after many years of little or no pain. The pain may be dull aching, cramping, or bearing down pressure felt in the lower abdomen or back. The pain tends to worsen with time and often begins progressively earlier in the cycle. Severe sufferers may have as little as one pain-free week out of each month.

The pain of endometriosis doesn't just occur at or before your period time. There may be pain during ovulation, during sexual intercourse (a sharp, shooting pain), during urination, or during bowel movements while menstruating. Other symptoms include infertility, abnormally heavy or irregular periods, and unexplained exhaustion and lethargy.

Who Is Most Likely To Suffer?

Ironically, endometriosis occurs most commonly in women who have otherwise normal, healthy menstrual cycles. Those women who have a history of non-ovulation, or of irregular and missed periods, are least likely to suffer from the additional problem of endometriosis. Women who ovulate regularly and postpone having children until they are will into their thirties are the most likely group to suffer.

Medical Treatment

If your doctor suspects that you may have endometriosis, the diagnosis is often confirmed through a hospital procedure known as laparoscopy. During a laparoscopy, a slender telescope-like instrument is passed into the abdominal cavity (either through a small puncture wound beneath the navel or through the upper vagina). This telescope allows the size and number of abnormal implants to be estimated.

Treating endometriosis medically can be a long and frustrating process. Depending upon your circumstances and age, you may be simply advised to have a baby! Of course this is not always practical or desirable (or even possible if you have already become infertile). Many women who do follow this advice find their endometriosis is greatly improved following the birth. Nine months of not ovulating tends to shrink the stray endometrial tissues. Pregnancy is not a panacea, though, and some women report no change, or even a worsening of their problems.

You may be given synthetic hormones to mimic the condition of pregnancy. These hormones (taken by mouth or injection over a period of several months) prevent ovulation and menstruation, and cause the same shrinking and disappearance of endometrial tissue as pregnancy does. This solution is far from ideal, however. Most hormonal treatments have a wide range of unpleasant side-effects, including weight gain, depression, acne, and nausea. One commonly used therapy, Danazol, causes masculinization as a side-effect—weight gain, voice deepening, and facial hair growth.

Although hormonal treatment provides relief from symptoms during the course of therapy, when the hormones are stopped (usually after about nine months), in many cases the implants become active again within a couple of months.

As a last resort in severe endometriosis, surgery may be suggested. Conservative surgery aims to improve or relieve symptoms by scraping away and removing as many endometrial growths as possible. Scar tissue and adhesions are also removed. Latest laser techniques allow endometrial growths to be vaporized without causing any harm to surrounding healthy tissues. Conservative surgery is often undertaken if infertility is a problem. If endometriosis is the only cause of infertility, between one-third and one-half of all women who undergo this surgery will conceive in the following three to six months.

A few women with long-term and extensive endometriosis may choose radical surgery as an end to their suffering. This involves removing the uterus and even the ovaries. Obviously, this is very traumatic surgery, and the physical and psychological dangers involved are not to be taken lightly. If your ovaries are removed, you will experience an immediate plunge into the symptoms of a premature menopause.

Natural Alternatives

Many endometriosis sufferers find that there are other, gentler, long-term treatments available in the field of complementary therapies. These include dietary change, the use of nutritional supplements and herbs, and having regular osteopathy and acupuncture treatments.

Diet and Nutrition

A holistic approach to the treatment of this disorder begins with dietary changes designed to increase your overall level of health. These changes include decreasing salt intake, and eliminating it completely for the seven to 10 days before your period. Spicy foods, animal proteins, sugar, tea, coffee, and alcohol are also dramatically reduced.

The bulk of diet consists of raw fruits and vegetables, along with whole grains, nuts, seeds, and vegetarian proteins. Fish and small amounts of chicken are also allowed. There is an emphasis on calcium-rich foods, including almonds, tahini, green leafy vegetables, sunflower seeds, hazelnuts, and bony fish. Calcium improves muscle tone and helps to reduce menstrual cramps so common in endometriosis sufferers. It is one of nature's most effective painkillers.

The British Endometriosis Society discusses several vitamins and minerals that have been found most useful for this problem. As well as calcium supplements, it suggests using vitamins E and B_6 (along with a balanced B complex supplement), evening primrose oil, and selenium.

Vitamin E naturally balances estrogen levels, and is useful for the hormonal imbalances common among endometriosis sufferers and also menopausal women. This vitamin also helps to keep the pelvic scar tissue soft and pliable, and consequently reduces pain from abdominal adhesions. Women with heavy periods often find that vitamin E reduces their blood loss.

If you have any problems with high blood pressure, start taking very low doses of vitamin E, gradually increasing the dosage over several weeks. Large amounts taken suddenly can further elevate high blood pressure. Beginning with 30 iu of E once daily, gradually increase the dose up to 600 iu daily (preferably with the supervision of your health care professional). If your blood pressure is normal, you can start with 100 iu twice daily, and increase your intake up to 600 to 1000 iu over a period of a couple of weeks (again, with medical supervision).

Because vitamin E is a fat-soluble vitamin (and is consequently stored in your body), it can be toxic when taken in high doses. It can also cause interactions with drugs you may already be taking. For example, digitalis medications taken for heart problems, or anti-coagulant drugs (used to thin the blood), are greatly enhanced in effectiveness when vitamin E is taken. If you are already taking any medications or have hypertension, please consult your doctor before beginning supplementation with this vitamin.

Vitamin B_6 has been a godsend for many women suffering from pre-menstrual syndrome. It helps to reduce such symptoms as headaches, exhaustion, irritability, breast tenderness, and abdominal bloating—all symptoms that endometriosis sufferers endure for weeks at a time. Vitamin B_6 is only one part of a whole complex of different B vitamins that work together. Always take this vitamin along with a B complex supplement.

Evening primrose oil is rich in gamma linoleic acid, necessary to keep your cardiovascular and nervous systems healthy. Endometriosis sufferers find evening primrose oil helpful for dealing with depression and fatigue (especially when they are the side-effects of hormone therapy).

Vitamins A, C, and E and the trace mineral selenium belong to a group of nutrients called anti-oxidants. Taken as a complex, this formula effectively reduces cell damage in many illnesses, including endometriosis. Selenium and vitamin E also have anti-inflammatory properties that help reduce the endometrial pain associated with inflammation.

Homeopathy

There are no remedies specifically indicated for endometriosis. Remedies depend upon the exact nature of the symptoms you present. Suitable remedies include those described in the entry on Dysmenorrhea found earlier in this chapter. As endometriosis is such a chronic illness, it is in your best interest to consult with a homeopath rather than to try to self-prescribe.

Fibrocystic Breast Disease/
Chronic Cystic Mastitis/
Mammary Dysplasia

Fibrocystic breast disease (FBD) can occur at any time of your reproductive life, usually between the ages of 18 and 50. It is the most common type of breast disease, affecting up to 50 percent of menstruating women at some time in their lives.

Fibrocystic breast lumps are benign, but have caused shock and anguish for many women when they discover their first "lump." These lumps can range from one tiny nodule the size of a pea to masses of painful lumps the size of a grape or even a golf ball.

Symptoms

You may have one or many breast lumps, which may or may not be painful. The lumps vary in size and sensitivity throughout the menstrual cycle. They are at their most painful in the two weeks following ovulation, and before menstruation. Firbrocystic disease is often worse during times of increased stress.

Causes

Every month your body prepares itself for the eventuality of conception. Your uterus thickens its lining in perparation for the embedding of a fertilized egg, and in the same way, your breasts begin to prepare themselves for milk production.

In the first two weeks of your menstrual cycle your body produces large amounts of estrogen, which stimulates the cells of your milk-secreting glands (along with the ducts that carry milk, and supporting fibrous tissue) to multiply. After you ovulate, your body secretes more progesterone, which sets off a process that eventually leads to milk secretion from the breasts. If, however, your released egg remains unfertilized, your body backtracks, breaking down these milk-producing cells. This "waste" organic material must be reabsorbed by your breast tissue (there is no outlet to the outside world as there is with the breakdown of your uterine lining). Problems occur if your growth of milk-producing cells has been over-enthusiastic, and/or if your breaking down and reabsorbing of these cells is inefficient. In these cases, the "waste" cells can form clumps and lumps, which you notice as painful, lumpy breasts before your period.

Fibrocystitc breast disease has shown clear correlations with over-consumption of dietary fats and caffeine—something that modern Western women should think about with their high average intake of fat and love of coffee, cola drinks, and tea.

Fibrocystic breast disease is itself a benign condition. However, there is a correlation between the incidence of FBD and increased susceptibility to the development of breast cancer. Women with FBD are three to four times more likely to develop breast cancer. You are especially at risk if you first developed breast cysts before the age of 20.

Medical Treatment

Usually the first stage of treatment is diagnosis. Your doctor will probably insert a fine needle into one of the cysts and draw off a little fluid or some of the cells. This material is analyzed to make sure it contains no cancerous cells. A breast mammogram is also often performed, even if the lab tests show no abnormal cells. There is no drug that effectively cures FBD, although some doctors prescribe the contraceptive pill to lessen breast pain.

If you have one or two largish lumps, your doctor may suggest surgical aspiration, during which the trapped fluid and dead cells will be withdrawn from the lump through a fine needle.

Diet and Nutrition

The first, simple self-help measure to undertake is to stop drinking coffee. Research clearly indicates a correlation between high caffeine consumption and fibrocystic breast disease. Often women who stop drinking coffee completely have a dramatic decrease, even a complete recovery from, FBD within six months. Even in those women who still suffer from FBD, banishing coffee seems to reduce their pain and discomfort during the week before their periods. So, start by substituting with caffeine-free beverages or herbal teas.

Do You Get Enough Iodine From Your Food?

If you are a vegetarian, not eating seafood and perhaps not using any kind of iodized salt, you may be lacking this vital trace element. Iodine is the dietary substance that your thyroid gland needs to manufacture the hormone thyroxin. If you lack dietary iodine, your thyroid gland may well be sluggish. Some experimental research indicates that hypothyroid women are more prone to developing FBD (see Iodine in Chapter 2 on nutrition for information on hypothyroidism).

If the above description fits, don't panic. Simply add more iodine-rich foods to your diet. A half teaspoon of good quality kelp granules each day should be enough to meet your requirements if you don't consume any seafood. If your breast lumps are painful, you may get relief from reducing your intake of dietary fat. There is a clearly demonstrated link between high saturated fat intake and the development of breast cancer. Cutting down on fat will lessen your chances of your FBD transforming into breast cancer, and at the same time will reduce the levels of discomfort you endure. Changing to a mostly vegetarian diet will also decrease your exposure to synthetic estrogens, which are used to fatten chickens and cows (and passed on to you when you eat them).

What of Nutritional Supplements?

The vitamin supreme in the treatment of FBD is vitamin E. This vitamin appears to work by rebalancing the abnormal estrogen/progesterone ratio common in women with FBD, and in so doing, reducing the cyst-promoting effects of excessive estrogen.

In clinical trials, vitamin E has been shown to reduce effectively the number, size, and pain of breast lumps in around 80 percent of women. In many cases, the FBD completely disappears within several months of regular vitamin E use. Effective dosage seems to vary from woman to woman, with some responding to as little as 300 iu a day, while others require up to 1200 iu a day. As there are contraindications for high doses of this vitamin, you are best advised to seek professional advice before starting vitamin E supplements.

Deficiency of the trace element selenium, which is only needed in tiny amounts (and indeed can be toxic if oversupplemented) is strongly implicated in the development of both breast cancer and FBD. Selenium supplements are available off the shelf in the U.S., but once again, seek professional advice before self-medicating. Garlic is one of the most note-worthy dietary sources of selenium—but not garlic grown in deficient soils!

As hormonal imbalance is often to blame for the development of FBD, nutritional supplements that are known to assist in the normalizing of female hormone production are also indicated. B complex vitamins, and in particular B$_6$, fall into this category, as does evening primrose oil (EPO). Balanced B supplements which supply up to 200 mg of B$_6$ a day have been shown to be effective, along with six 500 mg EPO capsules a day (taken in three sets of two capsules).

Homeopathy

- *Plumbum.* The whole of the breast feels hard and tender and there is often severe constipation too.

- *Carbo Animalis.* Indicated when the FBD affects the right breast and results in a clearly defined nodule which produces spasmodic pain.

- *Bryonia.* Hard, heavy breasts with slight heat but severe pain. The symptoms get worse at the time of menstruation.

- *Belladonna.* Hot breasts with hard, sore lumps which feel much worse with any kind of touch, pressure, or movement. The pain is shooting and darting in nature.

Herbs

The humble dandelion has long been respected for its liver-cleansing and detoxifying properties. It has also been shown to reduce the severity of breast cysts and fibroids. Dandelion is best taken as a dried herb or a tincture, rather than using one of the commercial dandelion coffees (which are processed and lacking in active ingredients). Use 10 to 30 drops of dandelion tincture daily, or two capsules of dried herb three times daily.

The lymphatic cleansing herb Phytolacca or Pokeroot has been tra-ditionally used as a topical application to decrease pain and lumpiness in breasts. This herb can be purchased already made into an ointment, which should be massaged into the breasts every day the lumps are present. Do not use this ointment if you are breastfeeding, as it is highly toxic if in-gested by a baby.

Packs

The age-old standby castor oil has a use when it comes to treating fibro-cystic breast lumps. Daily applications of castor oil packs have been re-ported to cure even quite serious cases of lumpy breasts.

Use a flannel or terry face cloth, folded over several times and dipped into castor oil until wet but not dripping. Put the cloth over the breast lumps and cover with a piece of plastic or cling film. Next cover with a hot water bottle, as hot as can be tolerated comfortably. Over this place a thick towel. Just sit back and relax for about an hour. When you have finished with your pack, you can wash the oil from your skin with a solution of water containing two teaspoons of baking soda. Try to use the packs every night, or at the very least three nights a week until your lumps have gone.

Acupuncture

In Chinese medicine the breasts are very much linked with the liver organ and meridian, and breast problems such as FBD reflect a liver imbalance. In particular, lumps in the breast indicate a stagnation or blockage in the free flow of the energy along this meridian. As the liver is a very volatile organ, greatly affected by stress and emotional disharmony, this stagnation of energy is worsened by stress. Many women notice that their breast problems are worse during stressful times in their life.

Acupuncture and Chinese herbs can be used effectively to restore the free flow of liver energy, and can dramatically improve FBD. This treatment is most effective during the early stages of the disease, when the breast lumps are still small and few in number.

Fibroids

Fibroids are non-cancerous tumors, or lumps, which develop in the muscle that makes up the walls of your uterus. You may have one or several fibroids, and their size can range from the size of a pea to the size of a melon! Fibroids are most common in women in their middle menstruating years. In adolescence and after menopause the incidence of these tumors is much smaller. It has been estimated that about one in five women over the age of 35 has fibroids (and many of them don't even know it).

Nobody knows what causes these lumps to develop, although their development and growth seem to be related to the hormone estrogen. During times of high estrogen production (such as pregnancy and when using the contraceptive pill), fibroids develop much more quickly.

There are four main types of fibroids, classified by the area and direction in which they grow:

- Intramural firbroids grow within the muscle wall of the uterus.

- Subserous firbroids grow outwards from the wall of the uterus, sometimes on a stalk.

- Submucous fibroids grow inwards into the uterus. These fibroids can also develop on a stalk, and can sometimes grow so long as to protrude through the cervix into the vaginal canal.

- Cervical fibroids grow in the wall of the cervix. These fibroids are rare.

Symptoms

It is not at all uncommon for a woman to walk around with a uterus full of fibroids for several years, completely unaware of her condition. Fibroids may be quite large (for example, your uterus may be enlarged to the size of a 12- to 16-week pregnancy), and still cause no symptoms at all.

Not all women are this lucky, however. If you have any of the following symptoms, fibroids may well be the cause of your problems:

- *Excessively heavy blood loss during your periods.* Your blood loss may be flooding or gushing, or you may pass a lot of clots. If your blood loss is very heavy and ongoing, you may end up with iron deficiency anemia, and symptoms of exhaustion, breathlessness, headaches, or dizziness.
- *Painful periods.* The pain can range from severe cramping (comparable to labor pains), to a dull, constant ache in your lower abdomen and lower back.
- *Any change in your usual bowel or urinary habits.* For example, you may begin to pass water frequently, develop frequent urinary infections, or have problems with incontinence. If your fibroids press on your bowel (a rather uncommon occurrence), you may develop constipation or piles.
- *Infertility.* Fibroids can sometimes make it impossible for you to implant and carry a fertilized egg. If the normally blood-rich lining of your uterus is thinned out over a protruding fibroid, any implanted egg will have difficulty surviving due to the faulty blood supply. However, many women with fibroids have no difficulty in conceiving and carrying a full-term pregnancy.

Diagnosis

If you suspect that you may have fibroids, visit your doctor or family planning clinic. Usually a vaginal examination, with palpation of the uterus, is sufficient to diagnose fibroids. Your doctor may also suggest an ultrasound scan of your uterus.

Medical Treatment

If you have fibroids, but no symptoms of pain or heavy bleeding, you can safely leave your uterus alone! You may well go through your whole life without your fibroids causing any problems.

If treatment becomes necessary, your doctor will usually prescribe some form of drug therapy, before suggesting surgery if the drug treatment fails.

Most likely, you will be prescribed a high-dose combined contraceptive pill to control your excessive bleeding. This is usually not particularly effective. If you are over 50, have a history of heart disease in your family, or you smoke, you fall into the high-risk category for using the pill.

If drug therapy fails to help you, you will be treated through more radical surgical means. In some rare cases, a D and C (dilation of the cervix and then curettage, or scraping, of the lining of the uterus) is enough to remove your fibroids. If this fails, you may be offered a myomectomy.

Myomectomy

Myomectomy, which involves removing the fibroids while leaving your uterus intact and functioning, is performed when your fibroids are still small, and your uterus is smaller than an eight-week pregnancy. The surgery is performed under general anesthetic, and following surgery there is still a 50 percent chance of conceiving and carrying a baby to full term. This surgery is by no means a panacea. There are complications, which can include hemorrhage, scarring, and adhesions which can affect your fertility or leave you with a legacy of back and abdominal pain and pain during intercourse. In around five percent of women, the surgery fails to correct the heavy menstrual bleeding.

If all else fails, the last resort treatment for fibroids involves a hysterectomy—that is, the surgical removal of your uterus. Needless to say, this is major surgery, and as such should only be contemplated if you have exhausted all avenues of treatment, conventional or alternative.

Natural Treatments

Natural treatment of uterine fibroids aims to increase the local blood circulation and lymphatic drainage of the whole pelvic region, including the uterus. This is achieved through regular use of castor oil packs, hydrotherapy, and osteopathic manipulation of the spine. Women who develop cysts of the uterus (fibroids) or breast (FBD) usual suffer from poor elimination and detoxification. For example, they are frequently constipated, often suffer from skin problems, and their kidneys and liver are often sluggish and inefficient detoxifiers.

First and foremost a dietary change is usually required. The diet should consist of an abundance of high-fiber foods, such as whole grains, and fresh fruit and vegetables. Blood- and liver-cleansing juices should be drunk daily. These include beetroot, carrot, garlic, and parsley; lemon and grapefruit juice; and apricot juice. All refined foods, white flour, sugar, saturated fats (including meat and dairy products), alcohol, coffee, and tea should be reduced as much as possible.

All the elimination systems of the body need to be encouraged to work more effectively. It's easy to think of only the bowel and the bladder as performing these waste disposal functions. In fact, your skin and your lungs are also important toxin eliminators. Encourage your lungs to work for you through deep breathing and regular exercise.

Your skin can take some of the detoxification load from your bowels and bladder if it is stimulated through regular skin brushing. After your shower or bath, brush your whole body with brisk circular movements using a natural bristled body brush.

Drink plenty of water, vegetable and fruit juices, and herbal teas to keep your kidneys functioning optimally. Your new diet, combined with regular exercise, will usually be enough to give a new lease on life to your lazy bowels.

Castor Oil Packs

Castor oil packs have been used by naturopaths for years as treatment for a wide range of internal and external ailments. As an external pack, they are used for breast and uterine lumps and cysts.

To make your own pack, fold a small hand towel several times and soak it in castor oil until it is wet but not dripping. Place it over your uterus (lower abdominal area) and cover it with a piece of plastic (such as a torn-up plastic bag). Wrap the whole of your lower abdominal area in a large sheet of plastic. Then place a hot hot-water bottle on top and cover the whole area with a towel. Lie down in a comfortable position and rest for about an hour before removing all your layers and the pack. Repeat this process several times a week and persevere for a couple of months if needed.

Hydrotherapy

The most effective hydrotherapy for uterine fibroids involves regular alternate hot and cold sitz baths as described on p. 192.

Herbal Help

A medical herbalist would treat you with herbs designed to improve your elimination, and blood and lymphatic circulation. They may also use herbal hormone regulators such as chaste tree, raspberry, and black cohosh.

Homeopathy

- *Belladonna.* The menstrual period is characterized by heavy flooding of bright red blood and clots. Any kind of movement or touch makes you feel worse.

- *Tarentula.* Heavy periods, accompanied by severe pain and restlessness resulting from multiple fibroids.

- *Aurum mur.* Heavy periods with a yellowish vaginal discharge throughout the rest of the cycle. The uterus is physically enlarged from the presence of the fibroids.

Genital Herpes

There isn't much good news about this painful and virulent sexually transmitted virus. There is no successful medical treatment, and no guaranteed effective natural treatment. Once you are infected, you carry this virus for life. Do yourself a favor, and focus on prevention.

Causes

The genital herpes virus is similar to, but not the same as, the herpes simplex virus that causes cold sores around the lips and mouth. The genital herpes virus is an extremely virulent virus, and can be passed on to your sexual partner even when you are not experiencing an acute attack. This means that you don't need to have a genital sore to be infectious. The virus can be active *before* a sore erupts, and for months *after* the sores have healed and disappeared. Condoms do not offer 100 percent protection against the virus, although they are an essential protective measure that greatly reduces infection rates for all sexually transmitted diseases.

Symptoms

Symptoms usually occur for the first time within four to seven days of contracting the virus. The first attack is usually the most virulent, with subsequent attacks becoming less and less painful. Women who have ever had oral cold sores (herpes I) previous to contracting genital herpes (herpes II) tend to have less painful attacks. An acute herpes attack starts as a tingling or burning feeling or an itchy rash in the genital area. The whole of the vulva may swell and become inflamed. Next you will notice a small patch of tiny fluid-filled blisters somewhere on the genitals (including the inside of the vagina and the cervix). These blisters burst to form grayish sores with red edges, lasting about 10 days before healing.

Pain is another feature of the sores, with a sharp burning sensation which is particularly severe when you urinate. Your first attack of herpes can leave you feeling as if you've been run over by a bus. The sores are often accompanied by a flu-like illness with fever and swollen glands. Once you recover from your initial attack, you will probably never experience such a severe attack again, although the chances of your suffering another attack are still high—there is a more than 50 percent likelihood of another attack within the next six months.

With herpes, the pain and inconvenience of the acute attacks is really only half the story. There are other, more serious, long-term effects to consider. Cancer of the cervix is on the increase, with an estimated 15,000 cases of invasive cervical cancer diagnosed each year. There seems to be a relationship between infection with genital herpes and future development of cervical cancer. Infected women are eight times more likely than non-infected women to develop cervical cancer. Female herpes carriers should make sure they have a pap smear every six months.

When it comes to having children, herpes causes still more problems. If you carry this virus, you are three times more likely to have a miscarriage, or a premature baby. Babies can become infected with the virus as they pass down the vaginal canal, with a 50 percent chance of infection if you have active sores at the time of the birth, and an 8 percent incidence of infection if you don't have sores at the time of the birth. For this reason, Caesarians are often chosen over vaginal births.

Medical Treatment
There is no cure for herpes; there are merely means of lessening the severity of the symptoms. The sore should be kept clean through bathing with a saline solution (lukewarm water with a little table salt dissolved in it). Your doctor will probably prescribe a topical painkilling ointment. It may also help to lessen the pain of urination by sitting in a bowl of warm water to urinate, or spraying the vulva with water as you urinate.

Complementary Therapies
After your first attack of herpes, subsequent outbreaks are most likely to occur at times when you are under increased stress. For example, if you are already fighting an infection such as a cold or flu, or when your immune system is hampered through stress and late nights, overwork, and poor diet. You can't change that fact that you have the herpes virus, but you certainly can have an impact on how frequently the attacks come to haunt you. Your job now is to attain a high level of wellness, and in so doing, to minimize the impact of the herpes virus. Often this involves a total change of lifestyle, incorporating regular exercise, stress control or medication, dietary reform, and nutritional supplementation. Following the advice offered in Chapters 2, 3 and 4 of this book is a good place to start.

Dietary Assistance
There is an amino acid (a building block of protein) called l-lysine, which may help to prevent acute attacks of herpes. L-lysine is antagonistic toward another amino acid called l-arginine. The herpes virus needs l-ar-

ginine to thrive. Consequently, by increasing your intake of lysine (and in turn inhibiting the absorption of arginine) you can create less favorable conditions for the herpes virus.

L-lysine is available as a nutritional supplement, but you can also increase your intake by including generous amounts of lysine-rich foods in your diet. These include potatoes and soy beans, dairy products, chicken, meat, eggs, fresh vegetables, and brewer's yeast. Foods to avoid (because of their high arginine content) include all types of nuts and seeds, raisins, brown rice, oatmeal, and chocolate!

You can also take lysine as a supplement, with one 500 mg capsule a day usually being enough to prevent herpes attacks. You are biochemically unique, however, and you may need higher doses than this. At the start of an acute attack the lysine dose should be increased to a 500 mg capsule four times a day. This should shorten the duration of the attack.

Between acute attacks, a nutritional supplement regime can be used to strengthen your immune system. This should include vitamin C (either calcium ascorbate or sodium ascorbate), zinc, and a high potency B complex. Look for a vitamin C supplement that also contains bioflavinoids, for increased absorption. It is easier to take the high doses required if you use a powder rather than a tablet. Calcium ascorbate is not suitable if you suffer from kidney stones. For a daily maintenance dose of zinc, 50 mg is sufficient. Take a balanced B complex supplement which provides at least 100 mg of each of the major B complex vitamins.

During an acute attack, your immune system has to work overtime, and consequently your vitamin C requirements skyrocket. Increase your intake to your bowel tolerance. To achieve this, keep taking vitamin C every two hours until you develop slight diarrhea, then cut back your intake slightly until your stools return to normal. Keep up this dosage until the acute attack has ended, before gradually decreasing your intake back down to your maintenance dose. You may be surprised just how much vitamin C you can take before you reach bowel tolerance—10 to 20 g (that is, 10,000 to 20,000 mg!) is not uncommon.

During an acute attack you also need an increased amount of vitamin A; 15,000 iu is a safe supplementary dose, with one halibut liver oil capsule containing around 4900 iu. Vitamin A is best taken after a meal containing a fat source. Because it is a fat-soluble vitamin, and consequently stored in the body, this vitamin can be toxic. If you are pregnant, don't use vitamin A supplements without first seeking professional advice, as this vitamin can cause fetal abnormalities if taken in excess.

Acupuncture

Acupuncture cannot cure herpes, but it is effective in reducing the length of an acute attack. Regular acupuncture treatment can greatly strengthen your immune system and greatly reduce the frequency of your attacks.

Topical Applications

Invest in a jar of 500 iu vitamin E capsules, and keep it in your fridge. Pierce a capsule and apply the oil to your herpes blisters to decrease the pain and itching, and to shorten healing time. Apply the oil two or three times daily. Alternatively, buy a good quality vitamin E ointment that contains at least 30 iu of vitamin E per gram of base. To this add some powdered vitamin C, and then apply to the sores two or three times daily.

Several herbs make useful topical applications. Pure aloe vera gel will reduce stinging and pain and itching, as will diluted calendula tincture. Slippery elm powder can be made into a thick paste with a little water and applied topically to soothe the area.

Herbal antibiotics such as myrrh, echinacea, and golden-seal can also be applied, either as tinctures (but be warned this may sting badly) or as powder mixed with water to form paste.

Herbal Medicine

Besides their usefulness as topical applications, certain herbs can be taken internally to boost the immune system and act as anti-virals and antibiotics. These include such herbs as garlic, echinacea, golden-seal, and myrrh. See a medical herbalist for advice.

Homeopathy

- *Graphites*. Used when there is an acute attack of painful, red, weeping blisters in the genital area. The weeping fluid is clear or yellow and causes itching, but no burning sensations.

- *Nitric Acid*. Marked ulceration of the genitals and/or mouth causing local cracking and tenderness. Especially useful for ulcers on the corners of the mouth.

- *Rhus Tox*. For blisters which cause a lot of itching and discomfort and local redness. Symptoms are made better with applications of heat and with movement.

- *Sulphur*. Used in chronic cases characterized by burning pain and secondary infection. Pain is very much worse with any type of heat.

Genital Warts

Genital warts are basically like any other warts on the body, only they occur in and around the vagina (or the penis). They are caused by a virus very similar to that causing warts on other parts of the body.

Genital warts are classed as a sexually transmitted disease, and are extremely contagious. They are transmitted through sexual contact, be it oral sex, or anal or vaginal intercourse. If you have intimate sexual contact with an infected partner, you risk a 70 percent chance of infection.

Although genital warts are very unpleasant to look at, their real danger is that they signal a greatly increased incidence of cervical cancer in women.

Symptoms

One to four months after your contact with an infected person, your warts will begin to appear. They can grow anywhere on or around the genital area and anus. They may resemble warts on any other part of the body, or they may simply look like rice grain-sized, dark pink bumps.

Medical Treatment

Treatment involves painting the warts with a potent tincture of podophyllum. The solution is left on for six hours and then washed off. A few days later the warts fall off. Great care must be taken not to get this solution on any skin, as it is extremely burning and will cause great pain.

In more severe cases of warts cryosurgery is performed to freeze the warts off. In the most severe cases, your doctor may advise laser surgery to remove the infected layer of skin cells.

Natural Alternatives

Warts are a viral infection, and your chances of developing them are greatly increased if your immune function is poor. If you do contract genital warts, you need to treat yourself internally as well as externally. This involves undertaking changes to strengthen your body's ability to overcome the infection, for example, nutritional therapy (see the immune booster program, p. 58), following a healthy diet, getting adequate rest and relaxation, and trying to avoid as many sources of stress as possible (see Chapter 4).

You will need to supplement with all the old faithful immune boosters such as vitamins C, A, and B complex, zinc and garlic. There are a number of topical applications recommended for treating warts. You may have to experiment a little, and if one local treatment fails, try another:

- Tincture of black walnut applied daily is said to dissolve the warts in a few weeks.

- Apple cider vinegar and cayenne powder can be mixed into a paste and applied to the warts. Cover with a sticking plaster.

- Apply tincture of thuja daily to the warts.

- Powdered vitamin C can be made into a paste and applied topically. Cover with a plaster.

Incontinence

If you can't go to aerobics because you can't stop your bladder from leaking when you do the jumping exercises, or you leak from the bladder every time you cough, sneeze, or laugh, then you are suffering from mild urinary incontinence. While this isn't exclusively a female problem, it is many times more common among women. This is partly because of the physical trauma caused during pregnancy and giving birth, and partly because of the natural aging process, which is greatly accentuated by the loss of estrogen after the menopause.

Causes

Stress incontinence is more common in women who have had a baby. During pregnancy, the increased abdominal load is held up largely by the thick sheath of muscle known as the pelvic floor. Obviously pregnancy places an added load on this muscle, and can cause stretching and weakening. If you fail to keep your pelvic floor well toned through regular pelvic floor exercise (kegel exercises, described in Chapter 3 on exercise), you may end up with a general sagging of your abdominal organs and a weakening of your urinary sphincter.

A stretched and weakened pelvic floor may not become immediately apparent, or may only cause occasional, slight leaking of urine. However, once estrogen levels drop after the menopause, weaknesses in this area tend to become even more evident. If you have had several children, long, difficult labors, a forceps delivery, large babies, or large tears, you are especially at risk. Other risk factors include being overweight (especially carrying excess abdominal fat) and having poor abdominal tone through lack of exercise. Temporary incontinence can occur following some traumatic emotional experience, such as a great fright or shock, or an emotional loss such as divorce or the death of a loved one. In these cases the cause is obviously psychological and emotional rather than physical. The incontinence usually resolves itself with time, as the emotional trauma is resolved.

Symptoms

Inability to hold urine in the bladder, especially during exercise or when coughing or sneezing. Symptoms can range from an occasional trickle to complete involuntary emptying of the bladder.

Medical Treatment

Medical treatment usually involves surgery to repair the sagging and weakened pelvic floor muscles. This operation does not offer 100 percent cure, and failure rates are usually around 10 to 20 percent. In some cases, incontinence can be improved through the daily use of a small rubber device called a pessary. This device is inserted into the vagina and stretches from the back of the pubic bone to the top of the vagina, acting as a sort of trampoline to hold prolapsed organs in place.

Alternative Treatment

If your incontinence is due to weakness of the pelvic floor, there are few real alternative treatments to try, besides a faithful adherence to performing kegel exercises daily. In less severe cases of stress incontinence, this can remedy the problem.

Infertility

Infertility is one of those infrequently talked about problems that you might think will always remain the concern of some faceless couple "out there." It is always a crushing blow when a man and a woman discover that they *are* that couple. The ability to reproduce at will seems to be a natural right, and it is something you may take for granted until the moment you discover that it is missing. In realty, this is a problem that affects approximately one in six couples, and 25 percent of couples in the 35- to 39-year age group. Also of concern is the fact that infertility is becoming a more and more common problem.

In the United States there is a sophisticated network of high-technology assistance available through private infertility clinics, for those able to pay large sums of money for their treatment. Your doctor can provide you with details about this technological assistance, if you require it.

The discussion below examines some of the less discussed aspects of infertility, and suggests what complementary therapies have to offer the infertile couple.

What Causes Infertility?

Because this is a resource book for women, the focus here is on female fertility. That is not to imply that infertility is most especially a female problem. Male infertility has become more and more common over the past few years. The last 30 years have seen an average 50 percent reduction in the number of sperm produced by men. In around 40 percent of couples who are unable to reproduce, it is because of male fertility problems.

You may be wondering at what point you should start worrying about the fact that you haven't conceived despite frequent unprotected intercourse. Statistics say that 80 percent of women having regular unprotected intercourse will conceive within a year. If you have been unsuccessfully trying to conceive for 12 months or more, it's probably time to start questioning your life style and general health.

To understand the myriad possible causes of female infertility, you first need to understand exactly how conception takes place. In order for conception to occur, there must be present a female egg (ovum) and male sperm. In healthy women, the egg is released from one of the ovaries every 28 days, with ovulation occurring about 14 days after the start of the menstrual period. Once the egg has burst out of the ovary, it begins a four-inch journey through the fallopian tubes to the uterus—a journey that takes four days to complete. Conception can take place at any stage of the journey, if sperm are present. If the egg is fertilized, it embeds itself within the thick, nutrient-rich lining of the uterus, where it begins its nine-month miracle of growth and development.

Problems can arise at any stage of this process. If you are not ovulating, there will be no egg awaiting the arrival of the sperm. If you are ovulating, but your fallopian tubes are blocked or damaged in some way (often as a result of pelvic inflammatory disease or endometriosis), the released egg may not be able to complete its journey to the uterus. Your vaginal mucus may be inhospitable for sperm, if it is excessively acidic, paralyzing the sperm and preventing them from completing their marathon journey to the uterus and fallopian tubes. Sometimes women actually develop antibodies to their partner's sperm, killing them off as though they were invading bacteria.

Major Causes of Female Infertility

- *Pelvic scar tissue.* Scar tissue around the uterus, fallopian tubes, and ovary, resulting from infections such as gonorrhea and pelvic inflammatory disease.

- *Fibroids.* Multiple large fibroids can distort the lining of the uterus and prevent implantation of a fertilized egg.

- *Cervical problems.* The cervix secretes mucus all month. At the time of ovulation the mucus changes, making it thin and penetrable by the sperm. Sometimes abnormalities occur with this mucus, causing it to stay thick and impenetrable all month, thus preventing the sperm from traveling up into the uterus and fallopian tubes. Alternatively, your cervical secretions may be too acidic, killing off sperm in large numbers.

- *Hormone imbalances.* Some infertile women have an abnormally short second half of the menstrual cycle. When the normal two weeks from ovulation to menstruation is shortened, the lining of the uterus cannot produce sufficient progesterone to enable the uterus to successfully embed a fertilized egg. Other hormonal imbalances, usually centered at the level of the hypothalamus (the master controlling gland in the brain), can result in failure to ovulate.

- *Nutritional deficiencies.* Deficiencies of vitamins A, E, B2, B5, B6, B12, folic acid, vitamin C, iron, zinc, magnesium, and essential fatty acids have all been implicated in female infertility.

So, if you are doubting your fertility, the first step is to take a trip to your doctor so that he or she can investigate possible causes of your inability to conceive. The initial investigation will usually involve testing your partner's fertility, as detecting problems in the male is a lot more straightforward than detecting them in the female. If your male partner is found to be all right, then it's your turn to be investigated.

Your doctor will try to ascertain that you are ovulating regularly, and that you have no physical abnormalities such as blocked fallopian tubes, tipped uterus, or uterine fibroids, which could explain your lack of conception. Sometimes your problem will quickly be discovered, but in many more cases of infertility, there are no identifiable reasons for the inability to conceive. It is for these frustrating cases of "indefinable infertility" that complementary therapies are able to offer some real hope. If your doctor tells you there is no reason on earth why you are not pregnant, it is time to start some serious self-examination, taking a look at your lifestyle, your stress levels, and your nutritional status.

Medical Treatment

If no physical cause of your infertility is discovered, your doctor will probably begin with a course of fertility drugs such as Clomid. This drug is especially used when your ovulation is infrequent or absent. Other drugs may be prescribed when there are hormonal imbalances, such as excessively high prolactin levels (in which case bromocriptine is prescribed), or when the functioning of the corpus luteum (the part of the egg follicle which secretes progesterone) is impaired (in which cases progesterone is prescribed).

Blocked fallopian tubes may be treated with surgery, although their repair is not always possible.

Self-Help for Infertility

Take a good, close look at yourself. Are you a picture of optimum health, with abundant energy, a strong immune system, and a relaxed and calm disposition? Or are you stressed, overworked, exhausted, and fighting off one cold or flu after another? If the latter sounds like you, your inability to conceive may be yet another reflection of your low level of wellness. Seemingly inconsequential factors such as your weight and the amount of exercise you have could also be part of your problem with conception.

It is well known that women need a minimum percentage of body fat to maintain regular ovulation and a normal menstrual cycle (usually around 18 percent). Frequent dieters or women who exercise obsessively may fall below this critical threshold, and find they are unable to have children when they want to.

If this sounds like you, start your self-help by cutting down on your exercise and allowing a few pounds to creep on to your more relaxed body. Your self-help starting point involves turning to Chapters 2, 3, and 4 of this book, and beginning to learn about and then applying a new, healthier way of living.

Optimizing your diet, beginning a program of regular physical exercise (as long as you're not one of the "over-exercisers" described above), balanced with relaxation and stress management techniques, will gradually improve your health and vitality. Think seriously about consulting an appropriate complementary health professional to help you with your "wellness" program.

I would strongly recommend at least one visit to a registered osteopath to rule out any possible structural contributions to your infertility. As all your pelvic organs receive their innervation from nerves running from the spinal cord, lower back problems may indirectly hinder the health of your reproductive organs and your ability to conceive.

Acupuncture and Traditional Chinese Medicine

Acupuncture and traditional Chinese herbs have also been responsible for the conception of more than a few miracle babies. Acupuncture effectively strengthens your vital force (chi), enhancing your body's ability to conceive and carry a child. A course of acupuncture for this purpose would involve a dedication to your treatment, with possibly months of ongoing regular treatment.

Traditional Chinese medicine placed great emphasis upon treating female and male infertility. A couple who failed to produce at least one son faced catastrophic social consequences, as without a son there was no one to make sacrifices to the gods. Without the sacrifices, one faced the prospect of having one's immortality cut off.

The treatment of female infertility through acupuncture and Chinese herbs is very much concerned with normalizing the state of the woman's blood, female infertility being viewed as a deficiency of blood, or a stagnation or blockage of blood.

Blood deficiency is often the result of a weakness of one or several of the major blood manufacturing organs—the spleen, kidneys, and heart. Traditionally there are several factors known to cause weakness in these organs, which are abundantly common in Western existence.

The heart and spleen function of blood production is very much affected by emotional disturbances. The heart cannot create blood if it is "longing" or broken (usually as a result of unhappiness in a personal relationship); and the spleen is weakened by continued worry, excessive thinking, or years of intensive studying.

Emotion aside, what you put into your body in the way of food also affects your blood production. The spleen function is seriously weakened by excessive amounts of cold foods and drinks. This includes physically cold food such as chilled, iced, and frozen foods and drinks, and also cold energy foods such as fruits and vegetables (especially when they are raw), dairy products, and fried foods. This is why traditional Chinese treatment of infertility usually also includes specific dietary advice.

Inexplicable female (or male) infertility can frequently be successfully treated through traditional Chinese acupuncture, Chinese herbal medicine, and dietary therapy. Treatment usually consists of regular, ongoing treatment over a period of time ranging from several weeks to several months.

Diet and Infertility

Your body cannot obtain a high level of health and readiness for conception if it subsists on nutrient-deficient, processed fuel.

However, your diet can affect your chances of conception in another and less considered way too—that is, through changing the pH of your vaginal secretions, making them "hostile" to sperm. Sperm need an alkaline medium to survive for long enough and stay strong enough to complete the arduous journey up through the vagina to the cervix. If your diet consists largely of acidic-type foods such as grains, meats, fish, eggs, nuts and seeds, coffee, and alcohol, then your vaginal secretions could well be acidic and inhospitable to sperm. This can be remedied by balancing your diet with more alkalinizing foods such as fruits, vegetables, and dairy products.

Nutritional Deficiency and Infertility

If you have been following popular nutritional advice to cut down on your dietary fats, you may have ended up with some unforeseen results.

The truth is, you need a certain amount of fat to stay fertile, in particular, essential fatty acids, found in cold-pressed polyunsaturated vegetable oils. Induced EFA deficiencies have produced infertility in laboratory rats, and although I'm not drawing a comparison between women and lab rats, it may be something for you to think about. Adding a couple of teaspoons of colf-pressed safflower or linseed oil to your diet, or taking three or four capsules of evening primrose oil, would be a sensible start to your "fertility boost" program.

The fat-soluble vitamins A and E are also particularly important for optimum fertility. Both help to maintain the health and cell integrity of the mucous membranes, including the lining of the vagina and the uterus. Vitamin E in particular has been labeled a fertility vitamin par excellence.

Once again, lab rats have shown that a diet sufficient in everything except vitamin E produces sterile rats. You also need more of this nutrient in your diet if you are increasing your polyunsaturated fat intake to boost essential fatty acids. Besides including plenty of E-rich foods (see chart on pp. 60-61), you need to supplement with 400 to 800 iu of alphatocopherol each day.

Some of the B vitamins have also been used successfully to treat infertility, in particular vitamins B_6, B_{12}, and folic acid. B_6 has been successfully used to treat women who were failing to ovulate because of excessive levels of the hormone prolactin. Supplementing with high levels of B_6 ranging from 100 mg to 800 mg a day favorably altered the women's hormonal balance, increasing their production of progesterone in the second half of their cycle. Within 11 months of starting treatment, 90 percent of the previously infertile women were pregnant!

This particular type of nutritional therapy is appropriate for women who fail to conceive because of a lack of progesterone being released in the two weeks following ovulation and before menstruation. When there is not enough progesterone, it prevents the lining of the uterus from becoming thick enough and nutrient-rich enough for the successful implanting of a fertilized egg. Interestingly, most women with this problem also suffer from marked pre-menstrual syndrome, another B_6 deficiency problem. A word of caution, however. These are very large amounts of B_6, and it is inadvisable to use this type of megavitamin therapy without supervision from a professional trained in nutritional therapy.

Clinical trials indicate that folic acid can also increase fertility in some women. It is unclear exactly why and how it works, but supplementing with 15 mg of folic acid a day facilitated conception within three months in women in clinical trials.

Mineral deficiencies are more common than vitamin deficiencies, particularly zinc and magnesium. Your body needs adequate supplies of magnesium to produce the female hormones estrogen and progesterone. If you display any of the magnesium deficiency symptoms discussed in Chapter 2, it could be that mineral deficiency is your problem. A balanced multi-mineral formula supplying at least 400 mg of magnesium a day could work wonders for you. The same supplement could supply you with the often lacking trace element, zinc.

Zinc deficiency is strongly implicated in both male and female infertility, and zinc is often successfully used to increase the numbers and vigorousness of sperm.

How Can Nutritional Therapy Help Your Partner?

If your male partner has some kind of fertility problem, such as a low sperm count or "lazy sperm," certain nutritional options can be tried.

One of the amino acids that make up protein is called l-arginine. This amino acid is available as a supplement, as well as occurring naturally in many of the protein foods you eat daily.

High supplemental doses of arginine, in the range of 4 g a day, have been shown to increase male fertility by increasing sperm count and mobility (making the sperm better swimmers!). To obtain this effect, arginine is best taken in 2 g doses twice daily, but should not be taken continuously for long periods of time. Instead, use it for two weeks followed by a break of one week before supplementing for another two weeks. If you have diabetes, *this supplement should not be used.*

Zinc, taken in supplemental doses as low as 50 mg a day, has been effective in improving liveliness of sperm, and increasing their numbers in many men.

Often male infertility is the result of "clumping" of sperm. When they bind together and are unable to move freely, they are obviously unable to swim effectively to reach the waiting egg. When 20 percent of the sperm clump together, the man is considered to be infertile. A study of 33 men with 30 percent sperm clumping showed amazing results by simply using vitamin C supplements. The men were each given 1000 mg of ascorbic acid a day for three weeks. At the end of this time there was an average 67 percent drop in the amount of sperm clumping, leaving only an 11 percent clumping rate.

Suggested Supplements for Male and Female Infertility

Female

- High potency B complex supplying 50 mg of the major B vitamins, to be taken twice daily with meals.

- 400 iu of vitamin E (alpha-tocopherol), to be taken first thing in the morning, or following a meal containing fat.

- Vitamin C and bioflavinoids; 1000 mg of vitamin C taken three times daily.

- Balanced multi-mineral formula supplying at least 50 mg of elemental zinc and 400 mg of magnesium in chelate or orotate form. To be taken between meals.

Male

- Multi-mineral formula (as above), supplying at least 50 mg of elemental zinc.

- Vitamin E (alpha-tocopherol); 250 iu to be taken three times daily.

- Vitamin C; 1000 mg of ascorbic acid to be taken three times daily.

- L-arginine; 2 g (2000 mg) to be taken twice daily, away from food.

Obviously, all the "wellness-enhancing" strategies appropriate for you can and should be applied by your partner, including stress release, regular exercise, and attention to diet and nutrition.

Often, inexplicable infertility is just another symptom of low levels of vitality and health, and when the general level of health is improved, fertility is miraculously returned.

Some General Fertility Tips

- Chart your menstrual cycle with the assistance of a natural family planning instructor. (Check your local Yellow Pages under "Family Planning" to find a clinic in your area, or ask a friend or a doctor for a referral.) This will help you pinpoint the exact time of your ovulation. Your egg only lives for 24 hours after you ovulate, so timing of intercourse can be crucial.

- Some sexual intercourse positions are better than others when it comes to making babies. Preferably use a position that allows deep penetration of your partner's penis (such as the traditional missionary position). Raise your hips slightly with a couple of pillows, and stay on your back for at least half an hour after intercourse to allow the sperm to make their journey without fighting the additional obstacle of gravity.

- Get your partner to put away all those sexy tight underpants and invest in some baggy boxers. Tight underpants hold the testicles close to the body, and in some cases this can lead to overheating and damage to the sperm, which need cool temperatures to stay healthy and viable.

- Think of how many times you have heard of couples who were unable to conceive, and so they adopted a child, and within a matter of months had conceived their own. This happens, and what it illustrates is the effect that emotional stress and tension can have on our fertility. When you are tense and viewing every sexual act as merely a means of achieving conception, you decrease the chances of this actually occurring.

Try to incorporate "making love" into a broader space of mutual sharing and pleasure. Remember the candles, the romantic dinners, the lounging in the hot tub (although not for too long—remember the effect of heat on the testicles!), the love and the togetherness. You may be pleasantly surprised what a difference it can make being totally relaxed when you have intercourse.

Homeopathic Help for Infertility

If you want to try homeopathy to help you overcome inexplicable infertility, it is in your best interest to consult with a registered homeopath. The homeopath will be interested in treating you in your entirety, not just the part of you which is "infertile." Consequently, to begin with, you may be given a deep-acting homeopathic remedy that is not especially indicated for infertility. Once your general level of health and vitality is raised, then a remedy more specifically aimed at the fertility problems will be indicated.

Menorrhagia

Few women discuss the amount of blood they lose during their menstrual period, so it is hard to know exactly what is normal and what constitutes excessive bleeding or menorrhagia. If you have to wear double pads, pass large clots, bleed for more than five days, or find that you build your life around never being far from the nearest toilet, then you are probably losing too much blood. The amount of blood you lose each month (be it heavy or light) should stay constant. If you suddenly start bleeding more heavily than usual, this could be a cause for concern, and you should seek medical advice.

Even if there are no serious pathological causes for your excessive blood loss, if left untreated, this ongoing loss will eventually affect your health detrimentally. When you bleed you also lose iron stores, leading to iron deficiency, anemia, and exhaustion.

Causes

Around half of all cases of heavy bleeding fall into the unexplained category. The other half are caused by a variety of pathological problems, such as:

- Fibroids
- Pelvic inflammatory disease
- Endometriosis
- Endometrial cancer—usually accompanied by bleeding between periods, too, and most common in post-menopausal women.

If you do not have any of these problems, your heavy bleeding may be due to:

- The use of an IUD
- The use of the injectable contraceptive Depo-Provera.

There are also a number of hormonal or physiological imbalances that can cause excessive bleeding. One of the most common is an under-activity of the thyroid gland (hypothyroidism). This tiny gland is, among other things, responsible for regulating the menstrual cycle. Around 30 to 40 percent of women with hypothyroidism also suffer from excessive menstrual blood loss. If this is the cause of your menorrhagia, you will most probably also have other symptoms of hypothyroidism such as:

- Dry skin and hair
- Lack of energy and easy exhaustion on exertion
- Tendency to gain weight easily
- Poor circulation and sensitivity to cold
- Depression and inability to concentrate properly
- Acne
- Recurrent infections.

If this sounds like you, start by performing the simple but remarkably accurate home thyroid function test described below. If your results indicate that you may have a thyroid problem, don't despair. While the medical answer involves long-term replacement of your natural thyroid hormones with a synthetic version (thyroxin), alternative therapies may be able to offer you a solution. Acupuncture, osteopathy, and nutritional therapy can each stimulate a return to normal thyroid function in some cases.

Test Your Own Thyroid Function

This test is most accurate when you perform it on the second and third day of your period. When you go to bed at night, place a thermometer by the bed ready for the morning. In the morning, as soon as you awake, take your temperature under your armpit. Leave the thermometer in place for 10 minutes. If your temperature is below 97.8F or 36.6C, you could well have a problem with your thyroid. Repeat the test the next day.

Medical Treatment

It is important that you have your abnormal bleeding checked out by your doctor. Even if you don't wish to use drugs to treat your problem, you must rule out serious problems such as cancer.

Your doctor may perform a pap smear and a D and C (dilation of the cervix and then curettage, or scraping, of the lining of the uterus) as part of his or her diagnostic tests. Having ruled out all the potentially serious causes of menorrhagia, you may be treated with hormones (estrogen, progesterone, or a combination of the two) to stop your excessive blood loss. To understand more about potential side-effects of hormonal treatment, see the chapter on the contraceptive pill.

As an absolute last resort, if all else fails, your doctor may recommend a hysterectomy. Make sure that you have exhausted all avenues of treatment (not just the orthodox medical way) before you resign yourself to this major surgery.

Nutritional Therapy

If you have ruled out all the serious stuff, and you're still spending a fortune on pads every month, then a change in diet and a few well-chosen nutritional supplements may be your answer.

Certain nutritional deficiencies will predispose you to bleeding problems. Your diet may be lacking in protein, for instance, as a result of following a poorly balanced vegetarian regime, or a "crash" weight-loss program.

Protein is used by your body to manufacture muscle, and smooth muscles play an important part in regulating and then cutting off the flow of blood from the tiny blood vessels lining your uterus. If your muscles are being given adequate protein through your diet, it may be that they are not getting the other nutrients they need to perform their contracting and bloodflow-damming function. Such nutrients include vitamin E, essential fatty acids, and the minerals calcium, magnesium, and potassium.

After each period, your body must "heal" the lining of your uterus, stopping the bleeding until your next period. This healing needs still other nutrients, especially vitamins A, C, bioflavinoids, and zinc.

In clinical studies, women with inexplicably heavy periods have in many cases been found to have extremely low blood levels of vitamin A. When their diets are supplemented with approximately 25,000 to 60,000 iu of vitamin A daily, their blood loss normalized (but don't use these high doses without professional supervision). Interestingly, a sluggish thyroid gland (another of the common causes of menorrhagia) will hinder your absorption of this vitamin.

Another vital "wound-healing" nutrient, zinc, has an interesting relationship with vitamin A. If you lack zinc in your diet, your absorption and utilization of vitamin A is hindered. Concentrate on including plenty of zinc-rich foods in your diet—whole grains, shellfish, pumpkin and sunflower seeds, and organ meats.

If your gums bleed easily and you also bruise easily, a deficiency of bioflavinoids may be partly to blame for your heavy periods. This substance, which enhances the absorption of vitamin C, is vital to maintain strong blood vessel walls. If you lack bioflavinoids (and vitamin C), the walls of your tiny blood capillaries become fragile and prone to rupture. Consequently, the healing of your uterine lining is also hampered. Vitamin K used to be routinely given to newborns at birth to lessen their chances of hemorrhage. This blood-clotting vitamin is not available as a supplement, but can be freely obtained from food sources such as leafy green vegetables, egg yolks, kelp, alfalfa, molasses, and fish liver oils.

Supplements for Menorrhagia

- A multi-mineral supplement containing calcium, magnesium, zinc, and iron. A chelated or orotate formula is preferable, to enhance absorption.

- Vitamin A supplement, such as halibut liver oil. Use up to 25,000 iu a day (five capsules).

- Vitamin C and bioflavinoid complex, supplied in the form of evening primrose oil. Take two 500 mg capsules, three times daily, throughout your cycle.

Herbal Help

Certain herbs are renowned for their astringent hemorrhage-stopping qualities. These include red raspberry leaf, shepherd's purse, cranesbill, cinnamon, beth root, lady's mantle, and periwinkle. An effective astringent tea can be made from equal parts of American cranesbill, beth root, and periwinkle. Use one teaspoon of this mixture for each cup of water, and let it steep for around 10 minutes before drinking. Drink the tea three times a day in the week before and during your period.

Alternatively, try using tampons soaked in astringent herbs to stem the blood loss during the actual period. Soak a tampon in a tea made from equal parts of wild alum root and white oak bark, with a little lobelia added. Press the tampon high into the vagina, so that it sits up against the cervix. Change the tampon every six or seven hours. As these herbs are not widely available in health food stores, you will probably need to obtain them from a qualified medical herbalist.

Homeopathy

If you suffer from a heavy loss of blood, and the length of your menstrual period is more than five days' duration, one of these remedies may help:

- *Aconite.* Along with the heavy, bright red and clotty blood loss, you will experience anxiety and faintness. There will be a red complexion and a general sense of agitation.

- *Nat Mur.* Heavy and prolonged periods also tend to be irregular. The sense of dryness of the vagina and other mucous membranes also results in constipation. Cramping lower abdominal pains are also present.
- *Sulphur.* Prolonged, heavy but irregular periods characterized by loss of thick, dark blood which irritates the skin and burns the vulva. There may also be burning-type pains.

Still other remedies are appropriate if your blood loss is excessive but the length of your period is normal (three to five days).

- *Belladonna.* Bright red, clotty, heavy blood flow which is usually early. Again, there is extreme sensitivity to movement or touch, and the complexion is flushed red. Often there is accompanying headache and irritability.
- *China.* Early, heavy periods contain black clots, and are accompanied by extreme tiredness and ringing in the ears.
- *Ipecac.* Extremely heavy, continuous flow of bright red blood. Menses are usually early and accompanied by severe, sharp pains in the middle of the abdomen. There is a sense of weakness and vomiting is common.
- *Nux Vomica.* Heavy, irregular periods that tend to stop and start. Colicky pains and constipation accompany the irritability characteristic of this remedy.

Acupuncture

Acupuncture has traditionally been used to treat a wide range of gynecological and menstrual problems effectively, including menorrhagia. Traditional Chinese thinking recognizes more than one type of heavy bleeding. Generally, your excessive blood loss may be due to "heat in the blood," or to a weakness of the chi responsible for retaining your blood within its vessels.

Hot blood produces periods with copious amounts of bright red blood that gushes from the uterus. The periods are often early, and there may be spotting during the rest of the month.

Quite often, this type of imbalance is accompanied by a tendency to headaches, pre-menstrual tension, and a general feeling of irritability and stress throughout the month. This is because of the liver imbalance which contributes directly to this kind of bleeding.

The heavy periods caused by chi deficiency are quite different. Although there is a heavy blood loss, it tends to be paler, more watery blood that leaks rather than gushes. The periods just seem to trickle on for days and days.

Whichever type of heavy bleeding you suffer from, acupuncture can most probably offer you effective help.

Osteoporosis

Osteoporosis literally means porous or honeycombed bones. With age, the bones decrease in mass and density as they are leached of their mineral and protein components, eventually resulting in weak, fragile bones that fracture easily and are slow to mend. In advanced osteoposrosis, the weight of the body itself is enough to cause spontaneous fractures of the vertebrae or hip bones. The simple act of sneezing may be enough to fracture one or several ribs!

Symptoms

Like heart disease, osteoporosis is one of those insidious diseases that you often don't know you have until it's too late. Sometimes, however, there are early warning signs such as a gradual loss of height, and a bowing of the upper back, known as dowager's hump. The clearest symptom of osteoporosis is a spontaneous fracture.

Causes

Your bones are living organisms that are constantly being remade as bone cells are dissolved and reformed. Bone is manufactured from several minerals, including calcium, magnesium, and phosphorus. Of these, calcium is the most abundant. Bones are not only made from calcium, but they also act as large storehouses for this mineral. At all times, your body needs a small amount of calcium circulating in the bloodstream. When blood calcium levels are low, stored bone calcium is released into your blood. If your diet is lacking in calcium or your body's absorption of this mineral is poor, large amounts of calcium will be released from your bones. Over many years, this continued pattern leads to osteoporosis.

Fragile bones are not exclusively a female problem, although they are much more common among women. Small-framed Caucasian women seem to be most at risk. Beginning in your twenties and thirties, pregnancy and lactation are often the start of your bone troubles. Your body needs large amounts of all nutrients, in particular calcium, during pregnancy and breastfeeding. Frequently, these increased nutritional demands are not met, resulting in demineralization of bones, even from this early age. This early bone damage is increased dramatically after the menopause, when you become much more susceptible to the action of the hormone that controls calcium levels in the blood (the parathyroid hormone). Consequently, more calcium is released from the bones than can be easily replaced by the diet.

However, osteoporosis is not just about your calcium intake. If it were, there would be a higher incidence of this disease among women from cultures with a traditionally low calcium intake, such as Asian and

African women. Ironically, these supposedly "calcium-deficient" women have a lower incidence of osteoporosis than Western women. This is because the development of osteoporosis is linked with a wide spectrum of different lifestyle factors over and above calcium intake. Western women are more likely to indulge in calcium-robbing dietary and lifestyle practices, including:

- Consuming large amounts of caffeine in the form of coffee, tea, and cola drinks.
- High phosphorous intake from cola drinks and red meat.
- Eating excessive amounts of protein.
- Smoking cigarettes.
- Overdosing on dairy products. Yes, the very food promoted as being the osteoporosis panacea is indicated as one of the causative factors for this disease when consumed in excess.
- Dietary nutritional deficiencies, including vitamins C and D.
- Over-use of pharmacological agents including antibiotics, antacids (indigestion remedies), anti-depressants, steriods, diuretics, laxatives, and chemotherapy.
- Drinking alcohol.
- Leading a sedentary life with little physical exercise.

Self-Help Treatments

When it comes to osteoporosis, prevention is certainly better than cure. Preventing osteoporosis involves a sensible dietary and exercise program, beginning in your early twenties. Prevention also involves more than swallowing a couple of calcium tablets each day (although this is an important part of the plan). Your bones increase in density until your mid-thirties. It is important to optimize this ability to build bones by supplying your body with all the raw materials it needs.

Not only do you need large amounts of the calcium-rich foods listed in the chart on pp. 60-61, but you also need to limit the foods that hinder the absorption or increase the excretion of calcium. A steak on the barbecue is almost a part of national identity, but too many steaks may leave you in a sorry state in later years. Meat contains 20 to 50 times more phosphorus than calcium. Since phosphorus and calcium must be balanced in the body, calcium is leached out of your bones to maintain the proper blood balance of these two minerals. Many studies show that vegetarians, and even vegans (who eat absolutely no animal products), have a much lower incidence of osteoporosis, even though their total calcium intake may be quite low.

If you wash that steak down with a can of soda, you are further compounding your troubles. A study from the Harvard School of Public

Health indicates that indulgence in soft drinks can cause bone damage. Out of 5398 women, the cola drinkers were found to be about twice as likely as non-cola drinkers to suffer a first bone fracture at 40. This is because, like meat, carbonated drinks contain large amounts of phosphorus. Try drinking mineral water or fresh fruit juice instead. Drinking a glass of fruit juice just after your meal will enhance your absorption of calcium.

Very few American women suffer from a lack of dietary protein. The very opposite is more likely to be the case. A certain amount of protein is needed for the absorption of calcium. However, too much protein can work against you by depressing the retention of calcium in your bones.

Too much salt and sugar also work against you, increasing the amount of calcium you lose in your urine.

To Prevent Osteoporosis

- Consume a diet high in fresh fruits and vegetables, supplying a large amount of vitamin C.

- Minimize your intake of animal protein, especially in the form of red meat, and maximize your intake of vegetarian proteins such as tofu, nuts and seeds, soybeans, and grains.

- Expose yourself to the sunshine *sometimes* to enable your body to manufacture its own calcium-fixing vitamin D. All that's needed is a few minutes' exposure each day.

- Include plenty of calcium-rich foods in your diet.

- Use a balanced calcium/magnesium supplement from your early thirties onwards.

- Exercise regularly, especially weight-bearing exercise.

- Use restraint when it comes to coffee and tea, sugar, soft drinks, salt, and cigarettes.

And What of Calcium Supplements?

Yes, calcium supplements do make a difference to your chances of developing osteoporosis.

The *New England Journal of Medicine* recently published a study of 301 post-menopausal women. Fifty percent of the group were on a dietary calcium intake of less than 400 mg a day, and 50 percent had an intake of 400 to 650 mg a day. Half of the women received a daily supplement of calcium carbonate or calcium citrate for two years. The other women received no supplements. The results were very interesting. The women who had undergone menopause five or fewer years earlier had rapid bone loss from the spine, even when they took daily supplements. The women who had undergone menopause six or more years earlier responded well to calcium supplements. Especially effective was the calcium citrate which slowed bone loss down to negligible levels during the two-year trial. In the group of women who received no supplement, those who had a higher natural dietary intake of calcium had the slowest rate of bone thinning. This seems to show that calcium supplements are important for post-menopausal women (from five years after menopause), and that the type of supplement used is important. (See the discussion on calcium supplements in Chapter 2.)

Exercise—The Other Important Preventative

Looking after your diet and using supplements is only half the bone battle. Making all these changes will be of only limited value unless you also get up off the couch and put on your walking shoes!

Weight-bearing exercise is vital to keep your bones strong and healthy. Gravity is essential for calcium to be fixed in your bones. Without the force of gravity, astronauts in space lose about 200 mg of calcium a day from their bones. Likewise, while you are lying at rest and your body is not fighting against the effects of gravity, calcification of your skeleton stops and calcium is pulled out of your bones. Every night while you sleep calcium is released from your skeleton and is lost in your urine the next morning.

Latest studies show that exercise can even reverse osteoporotic changes in the skeleton. The *Annals of Internal Medicine 1988* published a study comparing bone density in two groups of post-menopausal women. One group was made to exercise (walking or jogging) three times a week. After nine months of exercising, their bone mineral content increased by 5.2 percent; after 22 months, by 6.1 percent. Thirteen months after finishing the experiment (and stopping exercise) their bone mineral content had dropped back to just 1.1 percent above base levels.

The control group, who did not exercise, showed no increase in bone minerals.

To change your bone density effectively, you need to perform weight-bearing exercise at least three times a week for 20 to 30 minutes each time. Walking, cycling, and jogging are the most effective bone-protecting types of exercise.

What of Hormone Replacement Therapy? (HRT)

Long-term use of HRT is the modern pharmaceutical answer to preventing osteoporosis in post-menopausal women. While it is true that estrogen has been shown to dramatically slow bone loss, its effects are only present during the course of treatment. Once HRT is dicontinued, bone loss rapidly accelerates.

The question of the safety of long-term HRT use is still largely unanswered, with most of the current experimental findings based on studies of short-term use.

For more information on the subject of HRT and osteoporosis, refer to the discussion in Chapter 12.

Pelvic Inflammatory Disease (PID)

Pelvic inflammatory disease (or PID for short) is a term used to describe infection in the uterus and/or fallopian tubes. The infection occurs when pathological bacteria move up from the vagina to the uterus. The most commonly responsible bacteria is that which causes gonorrhea, but a range of other bacteria can also cause PID. However, current medical thinking is that in up to 50 percent of cases, PID is caused by a virus rather than bacteria. If you have a sexual lifestyle that puts you at risk of contracting a sexually transmitted disease, you are also at risk of developing PID.

Your risk is especially high at certain times when the usually tight opening to the cervix is dilated. This occurs during your period (which is why PID often flares up just after the period), and after childbirth, an abortion, or a miscarriage.

Another common cause of PID is the use of the contraceptive IUD, with 3 percent of users developing PID. The string hanging down from the uterus into the vagina provides a ladder for bacteria to move up into the normally protected uterus. PID can occur straight after the insertion of an IUD, as the cervix has to be artificially dialated to insert the contraceptive.

The long-term consequences of PID can be devastating. Women frequently become infertile as a result of this disease. Once the infection attacks the fallopian tubes, adhesions and scar tissue often form which block the passage of the egg from the ovary to the uterus.

Symptoms

The symptoms of PID range from mild to extremely fierce. If you experience any of the following symptoms, see your doctor immediately:

- Pain in the lower abdomen and/or back

- Pain during or after sexual intercourse

- Inexplicable pelvic cramps

- Any change in your menstrual cycle, and/or bleeding between periods

- Fever, nausea, swollen lymph nodes in the groin.

Medical Treatment

It is important to seek prompt medical attention if you suspect you have PID. Infertility is a high price to pay for wasting time in seeking treatment.

Oral antibiotics are always prescribed, usually for at least 10 days. Penicillin is often used, if the infection is still in the early stages. Bed rest is strongly recommended for several days at the onset of PID. Unfortunately, antibiotics are only effective against bacteria, and then only in about 80 percent of cases. If your PID is the result of a viral infection, the medical outlook may be pretty bleak. It is not uncommon for chronic PID to drag on, uncured, for months and sometimes years. In these chronic cases which fail to respond to drug therapy, the only medical alternative is surgery, to remove the progressively diseased tissue. It is in these chronic, so-called "incurable" cases that complementary therapies can offer some real hope of assistance.

Natural Alternatives

PID is an infection, and as such the "immune booster" nutritional program outlined on p. 58 is a vital part of your healing regime. High doses of vitamin E taken internally will help to prevent the formation of scar tissue, adhesions, and long-term irreversible damage. It is best to take vitamin E in one dose, before a meal or at bedtime. If you are taking supplemental iron, remember to take your iron and your vitamin E at least eight hours apart, so that they don't interfere with each other's absorption. If you have high blood pressure, or are taking medicine to prevent blood clotting, see your doctor before self-prescribing this vitamin.

Strengthening your immune system involves a lot more than simply popping a handful of nutritional supplements each day. The quality of food you put into your body each day also counts for or against you in your battle with PID. Optimize your diet by following the nutritional guidelines in Chapter 2.

Regular exercise has been shown to improve infection-fighting capability, while ongoing stress detrimentally affects the immune system. Regular relaxation in the form of meditation, yoga, tai chi, or whatever else you personally find relaxing is another vital part of your road to recovery.

Herbal Medicine

The plant kingdom provides some potent anti-microbials and antiseptics for the treatment of chronic PID. These include such herbs as garlic, echinacea, golden-seal, juniper, wild indigo, and yarrow. Two of the most effective are garlic and echinacea. Garlic has a recorded medical use stretching back 5000 years, and scientific studies have repeatedly shown how favorably garlic measures up against penicillin. While penicillin is only effective against gram positive bacteria, garlic is effective against both gram positive and gram negative.

The root of the coneflower (echinacea) contains a powerful antimicrobial chemical which, like garlic, has proven effective against both bacterial and viral infections. Native American Indians traditionally used this herb for treating a wide range of infections such as blood poisoning, septicemia, abcesses, and even salpingitis (PID). Echinacea has very low toxicity and can be effectively combined with other antiseptic herbs such as golden-seal, wild indigo, and garlic.

Golden-seal is a remarkable herb, with uses ranging from a digestive tonic and an astringent for hemorrhage to a powerful antibiotic. Its antiviral and antibacterial properties are so powerful that it ranks second to quinine as the most effective treatment for malaria. It is appropriate to use this herb for any kind of infection, and it has the added beneficial effect of stimulating the body's own immunity. Because of the chronic, lingering nature of PID, it is in your best interest to consult a qualified registered medical herbalist for treatment of this problem.

Homeopathy

- *Apis.* Particularly appropriate when the infection is centered in the right ovary or fallopian tube. The pain is severe and shooting and burning. You are irritable and restless, with little desire to drink.

- *Colocynth.* The pain is centered in the ovaries, is violently severe and may be accompanied by vomiting.

- *Lycopodium.* For less severe, right-sided pain centered in the ovaries or fallopian tubes.

- *Belladonna.* Violent, hot, restless, acute condition accompanied by high temperature and very red complexion. The slightest movement or pressure makes the pain worse. Pain comes in spasms and feels like stitches.

- *Lachesis.* For left-sided pain accompanied by a smelly, infected discharge and tenderness over the left ovary or fallopian tube area. Much worse with any pressure.

Pre-Menstrual Syndrome (PMS)

Women have been committed to prisons and psychiatric institutions under the spell of this condition. It is sometimes a cause of suicide attempts, car accidents, and child abuse. Its sufferers report a definite increase in relationship problems at a certain time of the month. It is called pre-menstrual syndrome, or PMS—a uniquely female ordeal endured by millions of women in this country and throughout the world every month. PMS has been recognized for hundreds of years in medical records around the world. In the stressful "rat race" existence of modern times, PMS has become an increasingly common part of being a woman.

Symptoms

You can suspect that you have some form of PMS if you suffer physical or emotional problems that appear to be cyclical and tied in with your menstrual cycle. Your symptoms will occur each month, sometime after day 14 (ovulation) of your cycle. They may last for anywhere from two to 14 days, disappearing on or just after the day you start bleeding.

The list of PMS symptoms is long and varied, with women tending to suffer from groupings of symptoms. For this reason, PMS symptoms are categorized under four main headings:

- *Type A.* A stands for anxiety. This type of PMS is most notable for its emotional symptoms of anxiety, irritability, and mood swings.

- *Type C.* C stands for carbohydrate cravings (you fall into this category if you would kill for chocolate in the week prior to your period!). Along with the sugar cravings come exhaustion and headaches (all symptoms of low blood sugar, or hypoglycemia).

- *Type D.* D stands for depression. This is accompanied by mental confusion, an inability to think clearly, and poor memory.

- *Type H.* H stands for hyperhydration, which is like waterlogging. You suffer from type H PMS if you swell up like a balloon, none of your clothes fit you, and your rings cut into your fingers when your periods are due. The fluid retention will also cause your breasts to swell and become very tender.

Women are unique, unpredictable individuals. Consequently, you may find that your PMS symptoms fall into one or a combination of several of these categories, although type A is the most common, accounting for around 80 percent of PMS sufferers.

Causes

Much remains unknown about PMS. What is for certain is that this debilitating affliction results from hormonal imbalance.

Type A PMS seems to result from an abnormal balance between the progesterone and estrogen produced in the second half of your cycle. If you produce too much estrogen, you will feel anxious, while too much progesterone leaves you feeling depressed.

Overproduction of hormones is not the only factor leading to imbalance. A sluggish liver, unable to break down these female hormones when they are no longer needed, can also contribute to the imbalance.

About 60 percent of PMS sufferers report type C symptoms. These "craving" symptoms are indicative of abnormal fluctuations in blood sugar levels. During the last week before your period, your body becomes sensitized to the main blood sugar-controlling hormone, insulin. Consequently, the sugar circulating in your blood is shunted into your body's cells rather too quickly. This results in rapid lowering of available blood sugar, with the familiar alarm signals prompting you to reach for yet more chocolate. If you are stressed, or nutritionally deficient (especially in the B complex and magnesium), this problem will be heightened. The quality of your diet has a direct bearing on these problems too. PMS C type sufferers have been shown to consume around 2.5 times the amount of refined carbohydrates as non-sufferers.

If you are a fluid retainer, and suffer from type H PMS, you are having problems with the hormones released by a tiny gland at the base of your brain called the pituitary. This hormone indirectly instructs the kidneys to retain water and salt, in turn causing your swelling.

While type D PMS only affects around five percent of women on its own, it is seen in combination with type A in around 20 percent of PMS sufferers. This depression is directly linked with a lack of estrogen production.

Medical Treatment

Allopathic medicine doesn't have much to offer when it comes to treating PMS. Tranquilizers may be suggested for severe anxiety and depression. Diuretics may be prescribed for the type H fluid retention and bloating. In severe cases of PMS progesterone therapy may be recommended (that is, using the mini-pill).

Self-Help Treatments

PMS can be effectively managed and in many cases completely overcome through a combination of motivated dietary change, relaxation, nutritional supplementation, and exercise.

Diet and PMS

Poor nutrition and low quality food contribute directly to the incidence of PMS. There are some foods that are known to worsen your problems. These include:

- Refined carbohydrates such as white bread, cakes, cookies, refined breakfast cereals, crackers, candy, and chocolate

- Foods that are high in fats, including dairy products and red meat

- Synthetic foods that are highly processed and full of chemical additives

- Caffeinated drinks such as coffee, tea, and cola

- Alcohol

- Salt and heavily salted foods.

If you suffer from PMS, restrict your intake of all these foods. In their place create a wholefood diet based on the principles outlined in Chapter 2, placing emphasis upon complex carbohydrates (whole grain bread, brown rice, whole grain pasta, whole grain cereals), plenty of fresh fruits and vegetables, low-fat protein sources such as fish, chicken, and vegetarian proteins, and cold-pressed vegetable oils (rich in essential fatty acids).

Nutritional Supplements

Nutritional deficiencies greatly predispose women to the miseries of PMS. For example, in clinical studies, women with PMS are found to have much lower levels of blood magnesium than non-sufferers.

In areas where the soils are traditionally lacking in this mineral, this deficiency is very common. In addition, many women who suffer from monthly bloating and swelling rely on diuretics for years on end. These same diuretics can cause the body to lose huge amounts of magnesium, which in turn greatly increases the severity of the emotional symptoms of PMS. When supplementary magnesium is used, moods are stabilized by its normalizing effect on blood sugar levels.

The B complex, and in particular B_6 (along with magnesium), are the nutrients supreme for PMS. These vitamins help normalize glucose metabolism, assist the liver with inactivation of hormones, and stabilize brain chemistry. B_6 deficiency is common in women. The low intake among many women is then further reduced by the B_6 depleting effects of alcohol, coffee consumption, smoking, and the contraceptive pill. The most common deficiency signs of B_6 are anxiety, depression, loss of sense of responsibility, and insomnia—all classic PMS symptoms.

Clinical trials going back as far as 1942 prove that B_6 supplementation significantly alleviates PMS problems, with dramatic mood improvement in around 85 percent of women.

Magnesium is needed for the proper utilization of B complex vitamins, and so if you're supplementing with one, you are better off supplementing with both. There are some excellent combined nutritional formulas designed specifically for women with PMS. These formulas provide a convenient and well-balanced starting point for your nutritional supplementation program.

Additional nutritional supplements can be added if needed, depending on which particular type of PMS you suffer from. For example, types

A and D PMS may need additional B complex and magnesium supplements; type B would benefit from additional zinc (to 50 mg a day), and vitamin C (up to around 3000 mg a day during the second half of the cycle); and type C may need essential fatty acids (evening primrose oil—up to six capsules a day in the second half of the cycle) and chromium supplement (200 mg a day) to help normalize carbohydrate metabolism and blood sugar levels.

Exercise Away Your PMS

Moderate amounts of exercise are a vital part of your "beating PMS" program. Simply going for a brisk walk several times a week, or taking up a sport like tennis, racquetball, or jogging, will quickly reduce your premenstrual suffering.

How Does Exercise Help?

In several ways. Through using your muscles regularly, your blood and fluid circulation is improved, decreasing the amount of fluid retention and swelling you experience. A good burst of aerobic exercise will leave you feeling relaxed and unwound, due to the flood of tranquilizing brain chemicals (endorphins) triggered through your activity.

Exercise also helps to regulate your carbohydrate metabolism and prevent the blood sugar fluctuations that are partly responsible for your PMS mood swings.

Relax!

It may sound ironic telling you to relax when you're feeling so strung out, but it is an important part of beating your PMS. You will probably have to *learn* how to relax, and the best time to start is during the two or three weeks when you haven't got PMS. The progressive relaxation and simple meditations outlined in Chapter 4 are an easy place to start.

Alternatively, you may find that yoga or tai chi, deep breathing, walking on the beach, or listening to beautiful music is more relaxing for you. Once you have found your particular key to relaxation, use it regularly, especially during your PMS days.

Thrush

Thrush is the common name for a type of vaginal yeast infection caused by an overgrowth of the *Candida albicans* fungus. It is an extremely common, and often infuriatingly stubborn, problem to treat. It is the cause of much female suffering, trips to the doctor, and sabotaged sex lives.

Causes

A healthy vagina has an efficient, self-regulating system that maintains a slightly acidic pH. This acidic environment prevents harmful bacteria from flourishing and causing vaginal infections.

Not all bacteria cause problems. *Lactobacilli* bacteria are a very important part of the vaginal regulatory system. The cells that make up the walls of the vagina store sugar (in the form of glucose), and as these cells are sloughed off, their sugar stores are released into the vagina. Sugar is a nectar for a whole host of undesirable bacteria and fungi. In a healthy vagina, however, the friendly *Lactobacilli* turn this sugar into weak lactic acid, thus maintaining an acidic environment hostile to the "undesirables."

If the acidity and bacterial balance in the vagina is upset, then thrush may become a problem. There are certain times of the month when your vagina naturally becomes more alkaline, and consequently more prone to infection. Around the time of ovulation, the vaginal mucus becomes slightly more alkaline, and during menstruation this alkalinity becomes even more pronounced.

When you are pregnant you may well experience maddening vaginal itching, resulting from the increased vaginal alkalinity caused by hormone changes. The contraceptive pill, with its hormone-altering effects, is often the cause of repeated vaginal infections. If you are under a great deal of stress or lacking sleep, your immune system is less effective, and also your vaginal pH alters, encouraging the proliferation of yeast infections.

A large percentage of yeast infections are the direct result of using antibiotics. A visit to your doctor for a course of antibiotics is frequently followed by a return visit for anti-fungal medication. Antibiotics kill bacteria indiscriminately. They are unable to kill the "bad" bacteria and leave the "good" bacteria unharmed. Once the *Lactobacilli* bacteria are killed off in sufficient numbers, the *Candida* fungus flourishes without constraint.

The delicate self-regulatory ecology of the vagina is easily upset by unnecessary intervention. Feminine hygiene products such as douches and deodorant sprays are both unnecessary and sometimes the cause of maddening vaginal itching. Frequent douching tends to dry out the protective mucous secretions in the vagina and upset the pH balance, leading to infections such as thrush. There may be brief periods of time while you have thrush when douching with anti-fungal substances may be appropriate.

If you are prone to vaginal infections, even the way you dress can worsen your problems. Tight jeans may look great, but they can play havoc with your health. Yeast infections thrive in hot, moist environments, and tight jeans which prevent air circulation around the genitals result in just such an environment. Likewise, nylon pants or panty hose prevent air circulation. Cotton pants and panty hose with cotton crotches help prevent yeast flare up. Sitting around the pool in a wet bathing suit provides the ideal opportunity for yeast infection to proliferate.

Diet can be both a powerful causative factor or an effective healer of vaginal thrush. A diet that supplies large amounts of refined carbohydrate (white flour, cakes, pies, white rice, crackers, cookies, sugar) will lead to an excess of sugar in the vaginal secretions, and a tendency to fungal infections.

Women who are iron deficient have a high incidence of vaginal infections. Read the section on iron in Chapter 2 on nutrition to decide if this may be one of your problems.

Symptoms

Itching, itching, and more itching. If you have thrush, you will know about it. The vagina, labia, and even the top of the thighs become reddened, irritated, and madly itchy. There is usually a yeasty-smelling, cottage cheese-like vaginal discharge, too.

Medical Treatment

If you see your doctor about your thrush, you will be prescribed anti-fungal vaginal pessaries or cream, and usually a cream to apply to the external genitals as well. Some of the modern "super bombs" need only be used for one or two days, although there is quite a high recurrence of infection with these short courses. The more traditional nystatin-based anti-fungals are prescribed for two-week courses.

While there is no doubting that these pharmacological preparations are convenient and usually very effective, they do have their drawbacks. Many women find that there is a high incidence of recurrence of their infections, usually within 12 weeks of using the pessaries. This is probably due to the fact that the underlying weaknesses or problems that caused the thrush in the first place are not addressed by simply using anti-fungals.

Complementary Therapies

If your life is a constant battle with this depressing problem, be assured that with commitment and perseverance you will be able to overcome chronic thrush using complementary therapies. Dietary change, nutritional supplementation, herbal medicine, homeopathy, and acupuncture all offer effective solutions to this problem.

Dietary Change

This is a really important part of your road to recovery. Immediately cut out all sugars and refined carbohydrates. Throw away the chocolate bars, cookies, and cakes! Even dried fruit and fruit juice are too high in sugar. Sweet fresh fruits and honey are also on the forbidden list.

Avoid all forms of dietary yeast as a supplement, or drinking beer, and make sure that your nutritional supplements are yeast-free. Most crackers contain yeast, too. Rice crispbreads and ryvitas are yeast-free, as are some heavy Pumpernickels.

Other forbidden foods include cheese, mushrooms, and melon (all of which contain some type of fungus that tends to aggravate thrush), wine, soft drinks, vinegar, and commercial sauces.

So What Can You Eat?

Don't despair, this is not a food-free diet! Build a diet around a wide variety of vegetables, with as much raw food as possible. Include plenty of fish, chicken, nuts and seeds (as long as they are fresh), lentils and soybeans, and whole grains. You can eat fruit in moderation, and some dairy products (excluding cheese).

Try to include plenty of unsweetened *Lactobacillus acidophilus* yogurt (that is, yogurt containing live cultures). This will implant the friendly bacteria into the bowel, and help control any overgrowth of *Candida* fungus living there. In turn, this makes cross-infection from the bowel to the vagina less likely.

Onions and garlic contain anti-fungal chemicals, and should be used daily if possible.

Nutritional Supplements

The list of supplements appropriate for this condition is long and expensive-looking. If you have problems with chronic thrush, you will probably be saving yourself money by consulting a nutritional therapist to prescribe for you.

The most useful supplements include:

- *Lactobacillus acidophilus* capsules. Nature's Way produces a range of specially coated high potency capsules, which guarantee delivery of the acidophilus bacteria to the intestines (rather than being killed by stomach acid on the way there).

- High potency garlic capsules or tablets. Nature's Way Garlicyn and Probiotics Kyolic are two of the most effective available.

- High potency B complex, vitamin C, and vitamin A, to strengthen the immune system and restore normal health to the mucous membranes lining the vagina.

- Caprylic Acid. Caprylic acid is a fatty acid found in the oil of coconuts and palm nuts, butter fat, and some vegetables. Caprylic acid is a useful part of a nutritional anti-fungal regime.

Nature's Way products market a complete nutritional program specifically designed to help combat vaginal thrush. This product is called Cantrol and contains garlic, *Lactobacillus*, caprylic acid, anti-oxidants, and the anti-fungal herb pau d'arco.

Local Therapy

When it comes down to douches or local vaginal applications, your options are many. One of the most effective, cheapest, and smelliest solutions is to douche with a homemade garlic solution.

Peel two smallish cloves of garlic and blend with a cup of warm water (in a food processor or blender). Leave the thoroughly blended solution to sit for five minutes before carefully straining through a piece of cheesecloth. Add another cup of water to the strained liquid. Soak a tampon in the mixture and insert high into the vagina. Leave the tampon in place for several hours. Change the garlic tampon three times daily. The remaining garlic solution can be used to splash the external genitals repeatedly.

A simpler (but in my experience less effective) alternative is to peel a garlic clove and simply insert it into the vagina. If you feel nervous about ever finding it again, you can thread a piece of cotton through the clove to use as a drawstring.

Using garlic, even the most stubborn cases of thrush usually clear up in a week to 10 days. A bathroom and kitchen smelling like an Italian restaurant is a small price to pay.

Tampons soaked with gentian violet and used in the same manner are also useful. Using a paint brush, liberally apply the violet to the external genitals also, twice daily for three to four days. Be careful not to get the violet on the floor or on your hands, as it stains dreadfully. Rubber gloves are probably a good idea.

A tampon soaked in *Lactobacillus* yogurt is another traditional naturopathic answer to thrush. The *Lactobacilli* change the pH of the vagina, making it less hospitable for the *Candida*. This treatment tends to be slower than the others mentioned. However, once your thrush has been cleared, it is useful to use the yogurt tampons twice daily for about a week. This normalizes the vaginal bacteria and acidity, and reduces your chances of reinfection. Alternatively, try inserting two capsules of Nature's Way Lactobacillus powder into the vagina. The capsules dissolve and are an effective way of delivering large numbers of friendly bacteria to the problem area.

Australian tea tree oil is powerfully anti-fungal and anti-bacterial. If you can find any, use diluted oil as a douche and to wash the external genitals to lessen vaginal itching. To make a douche solution, add one tablespoon to two quarts (half a gallon of water, and douche twice daily. As an external wash, simply add five or six drops of oil to a bowl of warm water. Standing in the bathtub or shower, squat over the bowl and splash the external genitals frequently.

For those times during your course of treatment when itching and burning drive you mad, the following local applications will give you some respite from your suffering. If you are at home, try taking a saline bath. Into a bath of tepid water, add half a cup of salt. Bathe for as long as comfortable, and try to encourage the water into the vagina. Salt baths can be taken several times daily if needed.

Calendula lotion can be applied to the external vagina, either full strength or diluted in water. Chickweed ointment is also useful to apply around the outside of your vagina to soothe the itching.

Simple Self-Help Tips

- Avoid tight-fitting trousers, nylon pants, and panty hose. Always wear cotton pants and crotchless panty hose or stockings and garters. Go without underwear whenever you can!

- Don't douche unless you have to (that is, when you have an infection).

- After a bowel movement, always wipe from front to back to avoid transferring bacteria from the anus to the vagina.

When you are under a lot of stress, your immune function is depressed and you are a lot more susceptible to thrush and infections of any kind. If you have chronic thrush, it may be partly due to excessive ongoing stress in your life. Relaxation, meditation, or tai chi may be an appropriate part of managing your thrush.

Trichomonas Vaginalis (TV)

Infection with the microscopic *Trichomonas* protozoa is responsible for this sexually transmitted disease, which affects about 20 percent of all women during the reproductive years. This protozoa is unknowingly carried in about 60 to 80 percent of all male urinary tracts and passed on to the female during sexual intercourse. It can only be transmitted when the penis comes into contact with the vagina, as this organism can't survive in the rectum or the mouth (and therefore isn't transmitted through oral or anal sex).

If your male partner is carrying TV, he will most probably show no abnormal symptoms. Occasionally a male carrier may feel a slight burning sensation in his penis after ejaculating. Once you are infected, you may harbor this organism for months or even years with no apparent symptoms or ill effects. Then one day, when the alkalinity of your vagina is changed through pregnancy, the pill, or excessive stress, the TV organism will be activated and cause mayhem.

Symptoms

If and when your TV infection flares up into a problem, the first thing you will probably notice will be a horrible-smelling, greenish-yellow vaginal discharge. This is usually heavy, thin, and frothy, and will make your vagina, labia, and inner thighs feel sore and inflamed. Having intercourse is definitely out of the question, and even passing urine can be painful. If you have a pap smear at this time, your results will probably be abnormal, but your cervical cells usually revert to normal after the infection is treated.

Causes

As in the case of all sexually transmitted diseases, at some point prior to your symptoms occurring, you have been infected with a pathological organism (bacteria). However, in the case of TV there are a multitude of other contributing factors that eventually provide a favorable environment for the invading organism to multiply forth and cause problems!

A healthy vagina is a wonderfully complex ecosystem that plays host to a variety of microbes and bacteria, all of which ordinarily exist in harmony with each other. Bacterial checks and balances ensure that no one organism proliferates to the point of causing symptoms of an infection. One of the most useful "friendly" bacteria living in the vagina (and the intestinal tract) is *Lactobacillus acidophilus* (the same type of bacteria is used as a live culture to manufacture *Lactobacillus acidophilus* yogurt). This bacteria helps to maintain the normal vaginal acidity of about four to five on the pH scale.

As the vaginal cells are sloughed off, they release their stores of sugar into the vagina. The *Lactobacillus* bacteria turn this sugar into lactic acid, thus ensuring an acidic environment to protect the vagina from an explosion of alkaline-loving bacteria such as TV and *Candida* (thrush).

So What Conditions Change Your Vaginal pH?

Stress of any kind, if it is excessive and long-term, will increase the pH of your vagina, making your vaginal secretions more alkaline. This same stress will also depress your immune system, reducing your body's ability to deal with the proliferating invaders. You are also more susceptible to vaginal infections at different times during your menstrual cycle. Around the time of ovulation, your vagina is bathed in a greatly increased amount of alkaline mucus, due to the effects of the higher estrogen levels that accompany ovulation. This copious discharge sloughs off large numbers of vaginal cells, which dump their sugar stores and increase your vaginal alkalinity. This alkalinity is at its greatest during the days of menstruation, as the menstrual blood itself is a sweet and alkaline medium. You may have never had a day's trouble from vaginal infections of any kind, until you become pregnant. During pregnancy the cells in your vagina store more sugar than usual, and consequently the vaginal pH becomes more alkaline.

The contraceptive pill with its artificially induced pseudo-pregnancy causes the same vaginal changes. If you take the pill, you are more likely to be bothered with vaginal infections.

Do you have a history of frequent antibiotic use and repeated vaginal infections? Antibiotics have changed the course of history with their profound life-saving capabilities. Sadly, however, these same wonder drugs have been the cause of months and years of chronic vaginal imbalances for many women. Antibiotics are indiscriminate killers, destroying friendly as well as harmful bacteria. One of the friendly bacteria to suffer is the Lactobacillus maintaining your vaginal acidity. Thus, your TV infection may become a problem following an infection and a visit to the doctor for antibiotics!

Frequent douching with anything upsets the vaginal balance, while the mechanical act of douching may itself injure the cells lining your vagina.

What you put in your mouth affects the health of your whole body, including the vagina. Too much sugar going in your mouth results in too much sugar being stored in the cells in your vagina, and too many vaginal infections. Diabetics, with their tendency to higher blood sugar levels, suffer from frequent vaginal infections, in particular thrush. Don't be surprised if your TV problem becomes apparent after a spate of sugar binging.

Medical Treatment

TV is treated with the powerful antibiotic drug Flagyl (Metronidazole). A seven-day course has a 95 percent success rate, with your sexual partner being treated simultaneously. Flagyl is an extremely strong drug, which can have unpleasant side-effects ranging from digestive upsets, nausea, and headaches to reduction in your infection-fighting white blood cells. If you are in your first three months of pregnancy, this drug must not be used.

Natural Therapies

The following suggestions can be useful adjuncts to the medical treatment of your infection. TV can be extremely difficult to treat, and there are times when even the powerful drug Flagyl fails to cure this problem. In these cases TV can linger as a chronic infection causing great despair and pain over a long period of time. In less serious cases, or at the onset of infection, TV can be effectively treated without resorting to Flagyl.

Follow the supplementary advice outline under the treatment of thrush, with the addition of 200 mg of zinc sulphate daily.

Local Applications and Douches
There are several different douches reputedly effective for treating this infection.

- In a pan boil up two teaspoons of powdered myrrh and two teaspoons of golden-seal, along with half a teaspoon of fresh ginger and one pint (two cups) of water. After simmering for 10 minutes, strain the solution and allow it to cool. Douche with this solution twice daily until all signs of infection are gone.

- Another TV douche is made by adding one tablespoon of tea tree oil to two quarts (half a gallon) of warm water. Use twice daily as a douche.

- The maddening itching can be treated effectively by external applications of soothing calendula lotion or chickweed ointment.

Further Reading

General Books on Women's Health

Airola, Paavo. *Everywoman's Book*. Phoenix, AZ: Health Plus Publications, 1979.

Barrow, Iris, and Helen Place. *Relax and Come Alive*. Heinemann, 1986.

Boston Women's Health Collective, *Our Bodies, Ourselves*. Penguin. NY: Simon & Schuster, 1984.

Lanson, Lucienne. *From Woman to Woman: A Gynecologist Answers Questions About You and Your Body*. NY: Knopf, 1975.

Madaras, Lynda, and Jane Patterson. *Womancare: A Gynaecological Guide to Your Body*. NY: Avon, 1981.

Padus, Emrika. *The Woman's Encyclopedia of Health and Natural Healing*. Emmaus, PA: Rodale Press, 1981.

Nutrition

Coory, D. *New Zealand Nutrition and Your Health*. David Coory, 1988.

Haas, Elson M. *Staying Healthy With Nutrition*. Millbrae, CA: Celestial Arts, 1992.

Quillin, Patrick. *Healing Nutrients: The People's Guide To Using C*. NY: Penguin, 1989.

Reuben, Carolyn, and Joan Priestley. *What Every Women Should Know About Vitamins, Minerals, Enzymes, & Ameno Acids*. San Francisco: Thorsons, 1991.

Exercise

Pontefract, R. *Feel Fit, Come Alive*. Oxford University Press, 1979.

Reed Gach, Michael. *The Bum Back Book: Acupressure Self-Help Back Care for Relieving Tension & Pain*. Berkeley, CA: Celestial Arts, 1983.

Soloman, H. *The Exercise Myth*. San Diego, CA: Harcourt Brace Jovanich, 1984.

Alternative Therapies and Remedies

Fischer-Rizzi, Susanne. *Complete Aromatherapy Handbook Essential Oils for Radiant Health.* NY: Sterling Publishing, 1992.

Hoffmann, David. *The Holistic Herbal: A Herbal Celebrating the Wholeness of Life (2nd ed.).* Rockport, MA: Element, 1992.

Kloss, Jethro. *Back to Eden (2nd ed.).* Loma Linda, CA: Back to Eden Books, 1992.

Mills, Simon. *Alternatives in Healing.* NY: Macmillian, 1988.

Nissim, Rina. *Natural Healing in Gynecology.* Pandora, 1984.

Smith, Trevor. *Homeopathic Medicine for Women.* Rochester, VT: Healing Arts Press, 1989.

Stein, Diane. *The Natural Remedy Book for Women.* Freedom, CA: Crossing Press, 1992.

Tierra, Lesley. *The Herbs of Life: Health & Healing Using Western & Chinese Techniques.* Freedom, CA: Crossing Press, 1992

Van Stratem, Michael. *The Complete Natural Health Consultant.* Angus and Robertson, 1988.

Vogel, H. *The Natural Doctor.* Mainstream Publishing, 1989.

Westcott, Patsy, and Leyardia Black. *Alternative Health Care for Women: A Women's Guide to Self-Help Treatments and Natural Therapies.* Collins, 1987.

Contraception

Grant, E. *The Bitter Pill.* Elm Tree Books, 1985.

Clubb, E., and J. Knight. *Fertility: A Comprehensive Guide to Natural Family Planning.* UK: David and Charles, 1987.

Pregnancy and Childbirth

Lim, Robin. *After the Baby's Birth: A Woman's Way to Wellness.* Berkeley, CA: Celestial Arts, 1991.

Tannerhouse, Norra. *Pre-Conceptions.* Chicago: Contemporary Books, 1988.

Menopause

Budoff, Penny Wise. *No More Hot Flashes and Other Good News.* NY: Putnam, 1983.

Kahn, Ada, and Linda Hughey Holt. *Menopause: The Best Years of Your Life?* Bloomsbury, 1987.

Lark, Susan M. *The Menopause Self-Help Book: A Woman's Guide To Feeling Wonderful for the Second Half of Her Life.* Berkeley, CA: Celestial Arts, 1990.

Loney, Sandra. *The Menopause Industry: How the Medical Establishment Exploits Women.* NY: Penguin Books, 1991.

Mackenzie, Raewyn. *Menopause.* Reed Methuen, 1985.

Potter, Leteia. *Women in Mid Life.* New Women's Press, 1991.

Reitz, Rosetta. *Menopause—A Positive Approach.* NY: Penguin Books, 1979.

Shreeve, C. *Overcoming Menopause Naturally.* Century Arrow, 1986.

Pre-Menstrual Syndrome

Duchworth, Helen. *Premenstrual Syndrome: Your Options.* New Women's Press, 1989.

Hecate Women's Health Collective. *Premenstrual Experience.* Reed, 1984.

Lark, Susan M. *PMS Self-Help Book.* Berkeley, CA: Celestial Arts, 1984.

Index